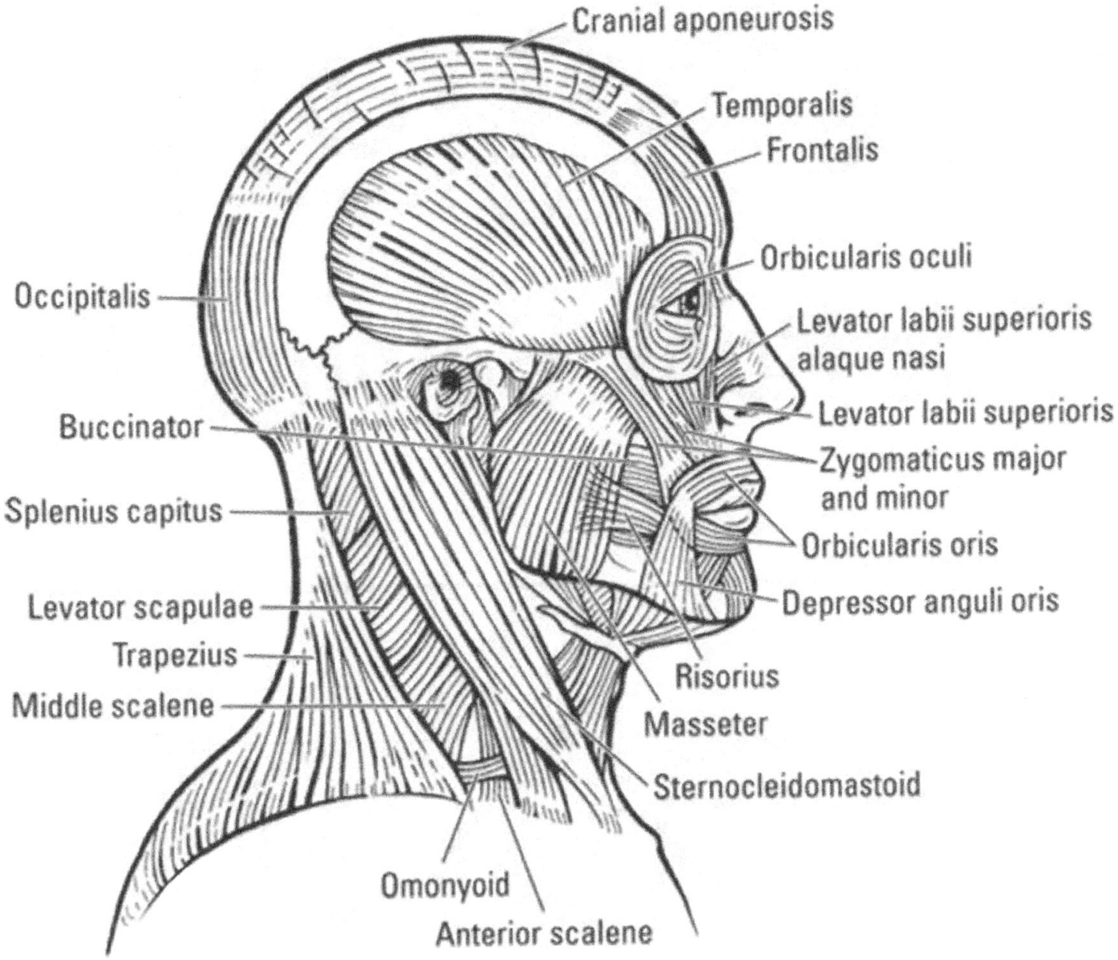
Cranial aponeurosis
Temporalis
Frontalis
Orbicularis oculi
Occipitalis
Levator labii superioris alaque nasi
Levator labii superioris
Buccinator
Zygomaticus major and minor
Splenius capitus
Orbicularis oris
Levator scapulae
Depressor anguli oris
Trapezius
Risorius
Middle scalene
Masseter
Sternocleidomastoid
Omonyoid
Anterior scalene

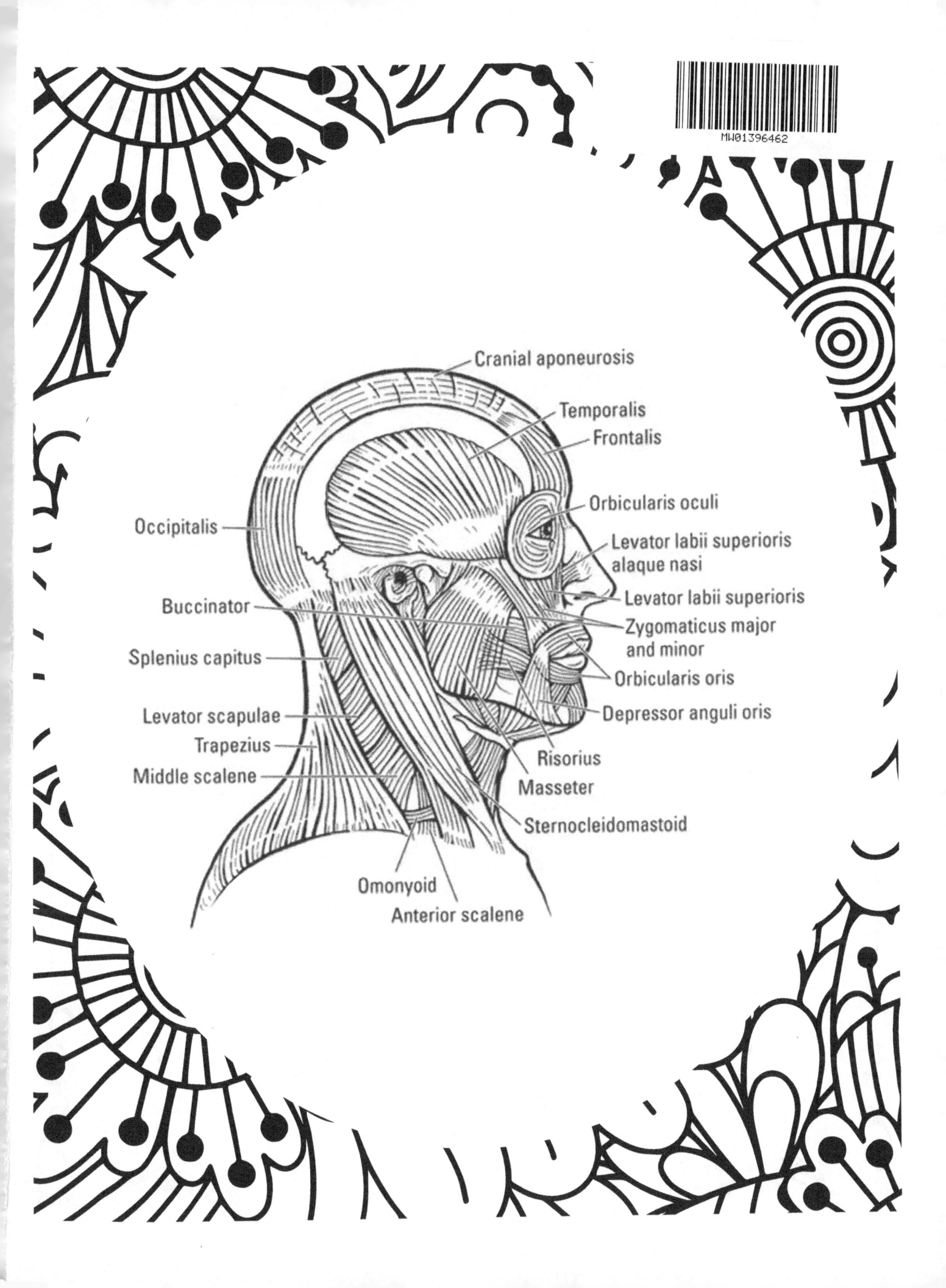

This Book Belongs To

Muscle Names

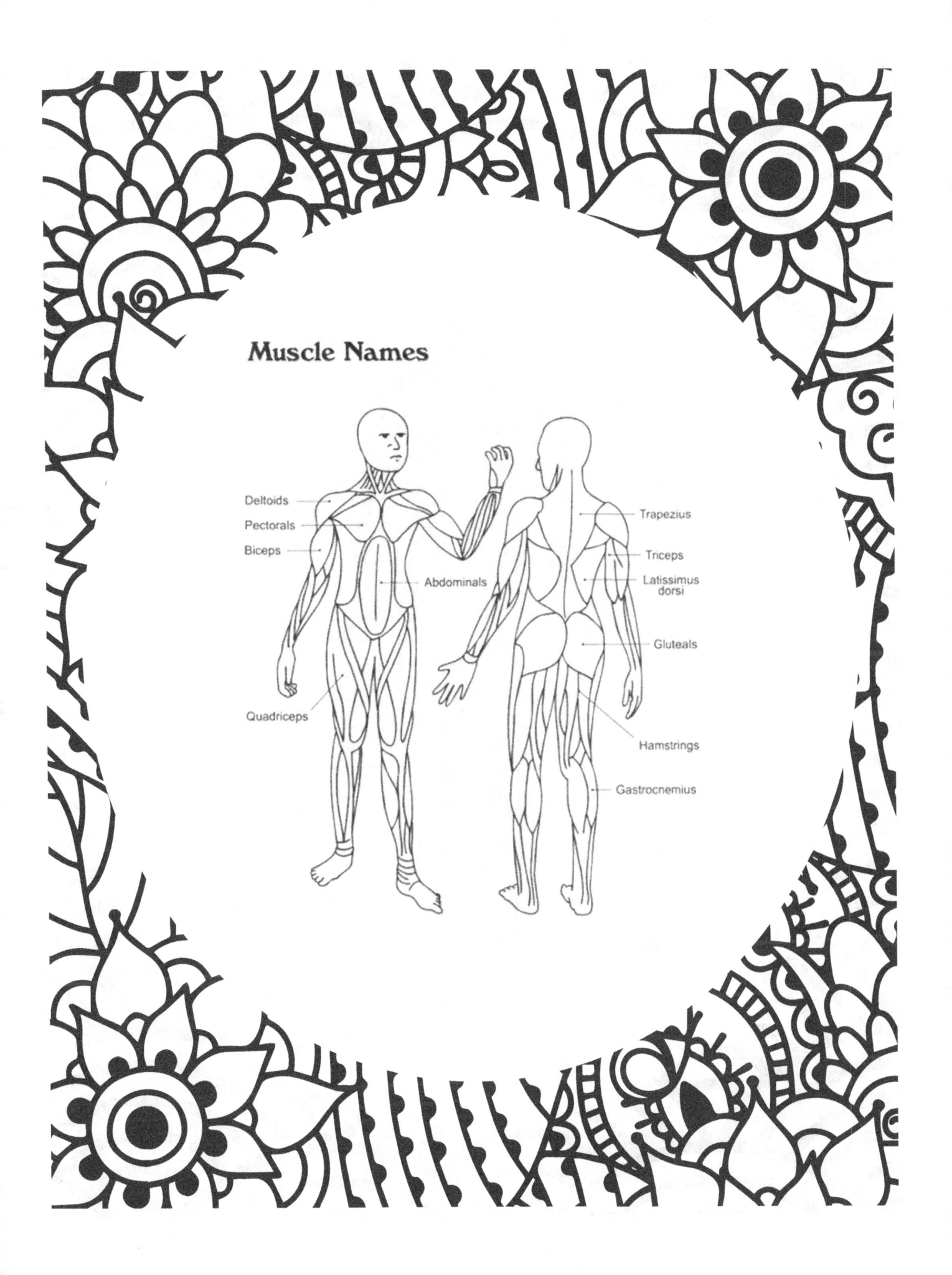

- Deltoids
- Pectorals
- Biceps
- Abdominals
- Quadriceps
- Trapezius
- Triceps
- Latissimus dorsi
- Gluteals
- Hamstrings
- Gastrocnemius

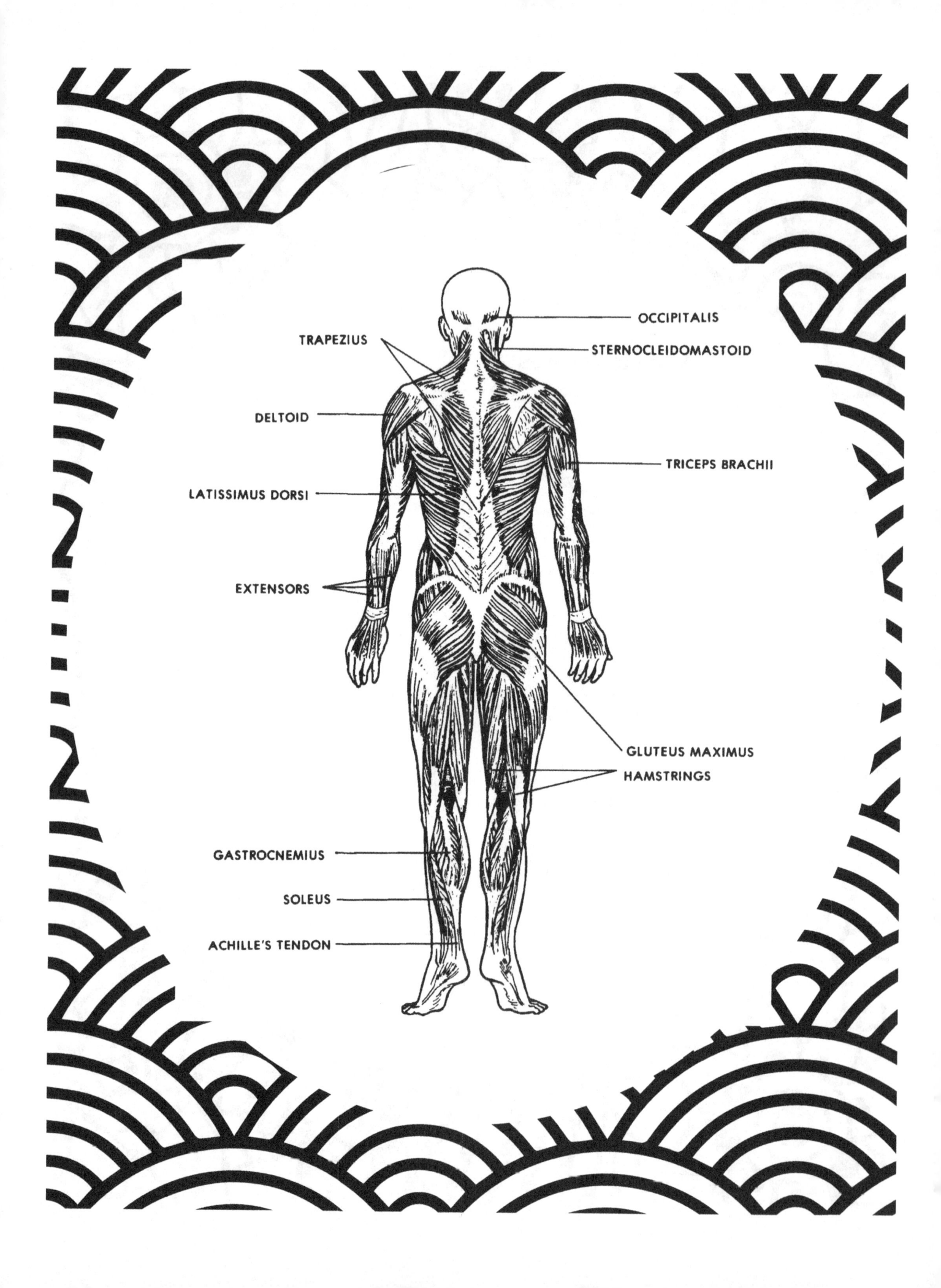

- OCCIPITALIS
- TRAPEZIUS
- STERNOCLEIDOMASTOID
- DELTOID
- TRICEPS BRACHII
- LATISSIMUS DORSI
- EXTENSORS
- GLUTEUS MAXIMUS
- HAMSTRINGS
- GASTROCNEMIUS
- SOLEUS
- ACHILLE'S TENDON

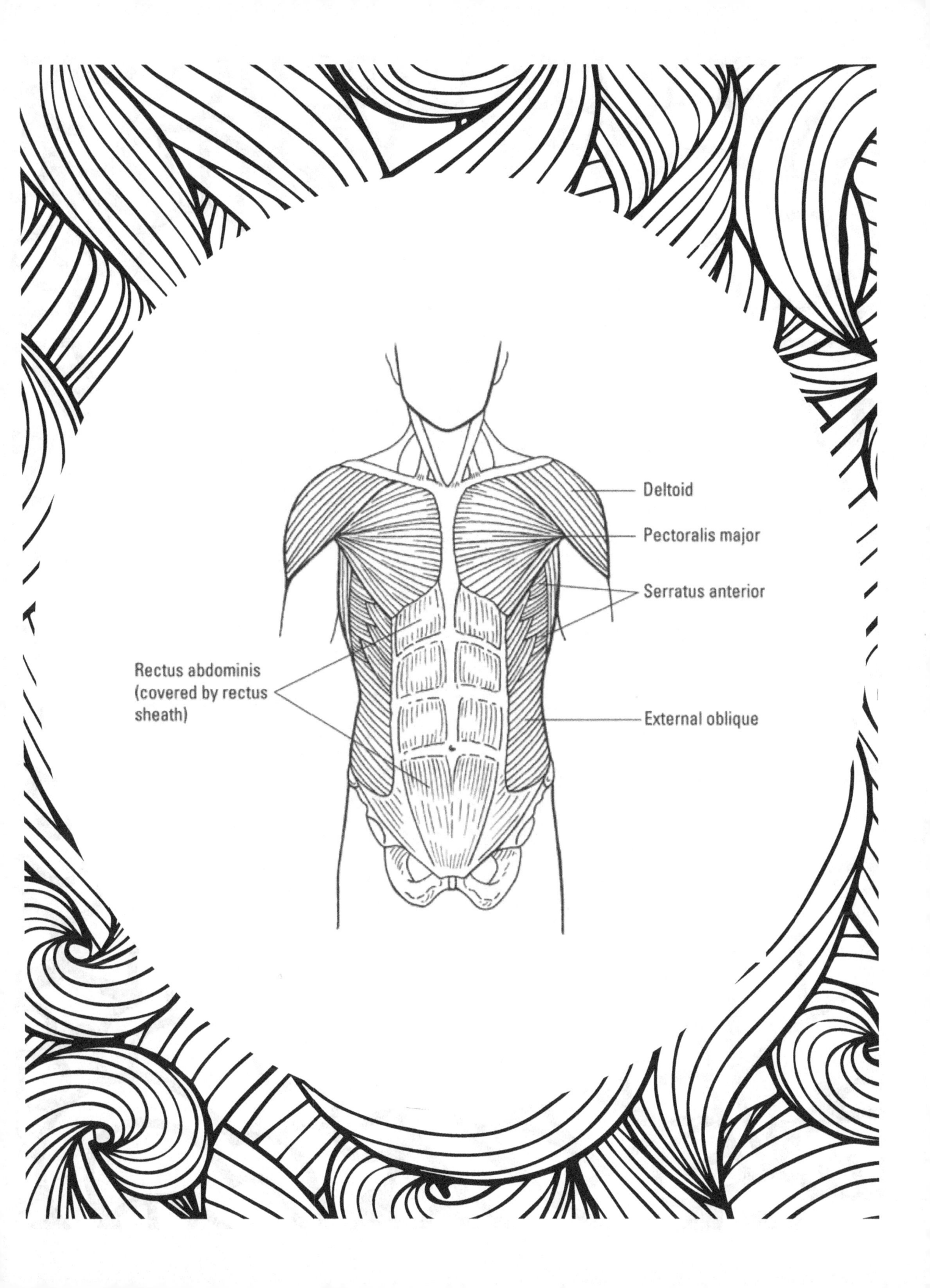

- Deltoid
- Pectoralis major
- Serratus anterior
- Rectus abdominis (covered by rectus sheath)
- External oblique

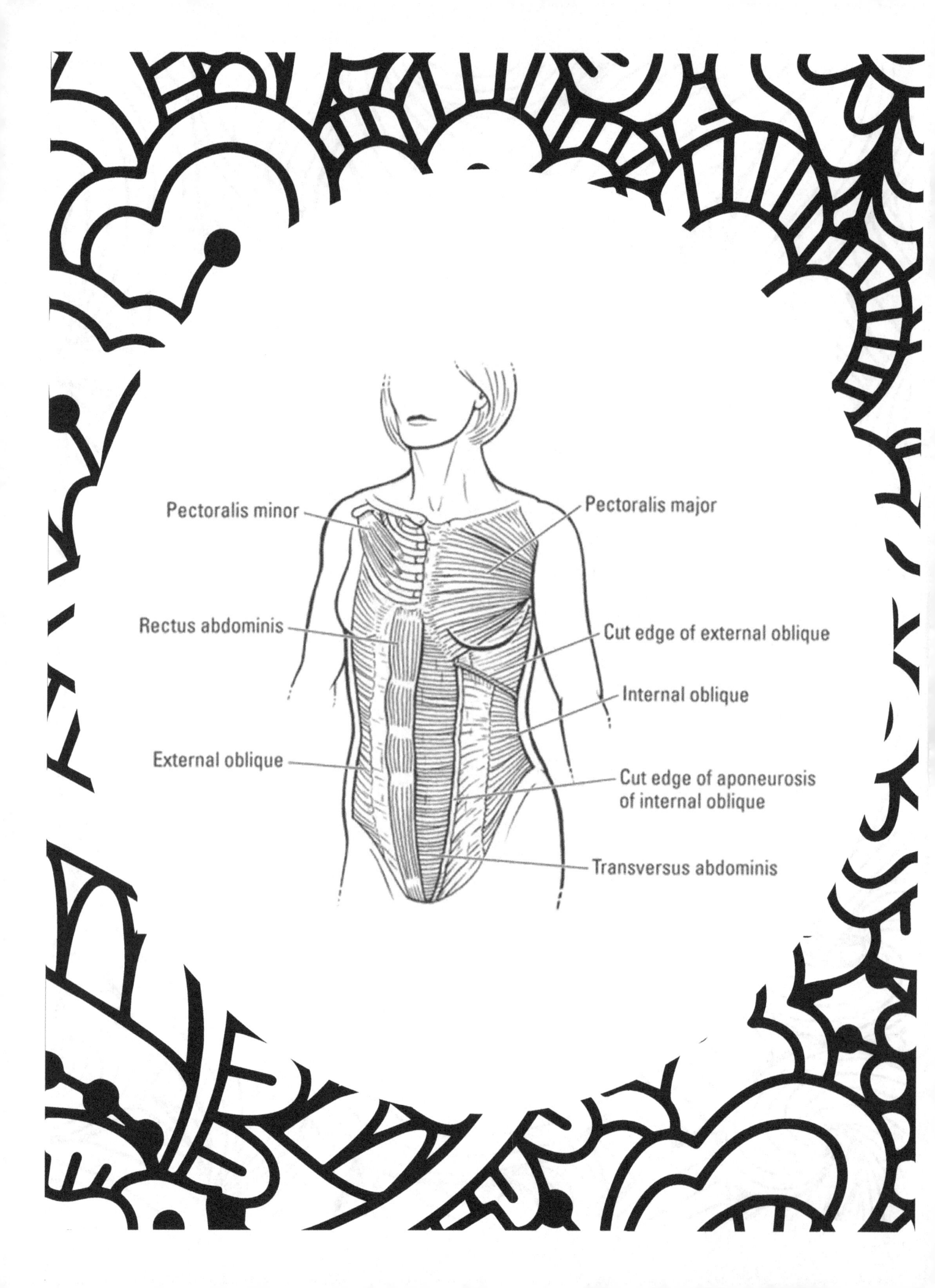

- Pectoralis minor
- Pectoralis major
- Rectus abdominis
- Cut edge of external oblique
- Internal oblique
- External oblique
- Cut edge of aponeurosis of internal oblique
- Transversus abdominis

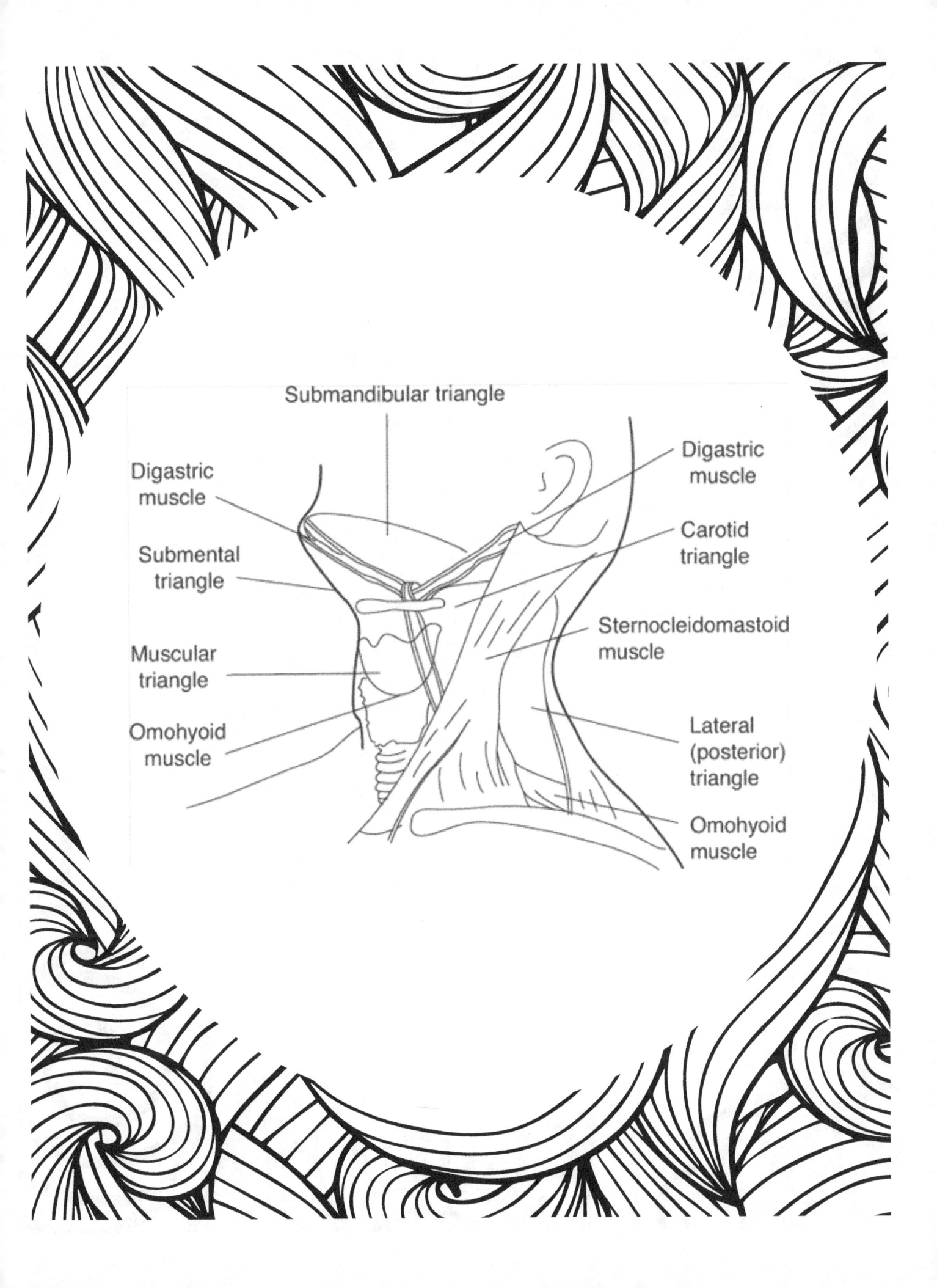

- Submandibular triangle
- Digastric muscle
- Submental triangle
- Muscular triangle
- Omohyoid muscle
- Digastric muscle
- Carotid triangle
- Sternocleidomastoid muscle
- Lateral (posterior) triangle
- Omohyoid muscle

The Shoulder Joint

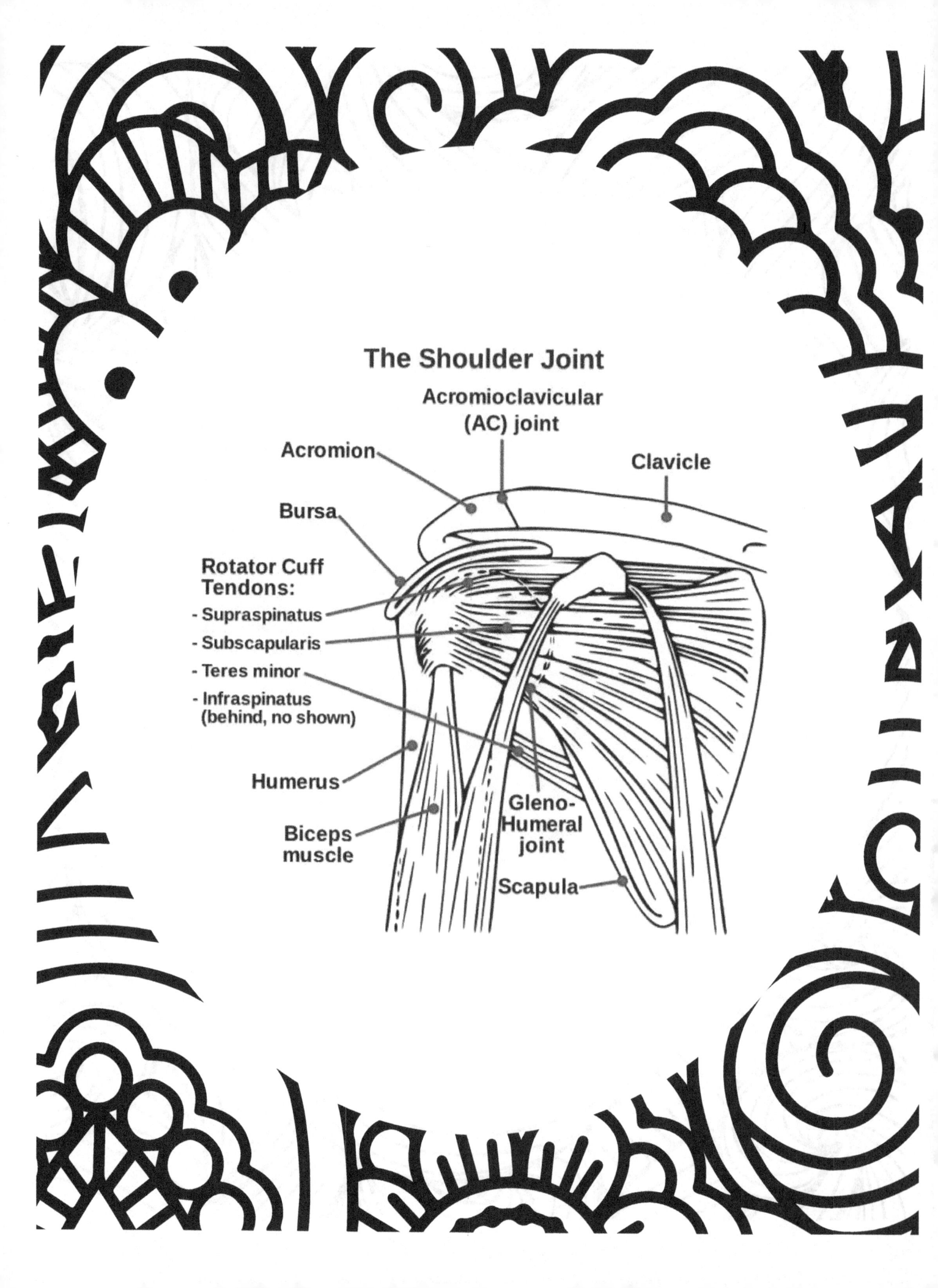

- Acromioclavicular (AC) joint
- Acromion
- Clavicle
- Bursa
- Rotator Cuff Tendons:
  - Supraspinatus
  - Subscapularis
  - Teres minor
  - Infraspinatus (behind, no shown)
- Humerus
- Biceps muscle
- Gleno-Humeral joint
- Scapula

Base

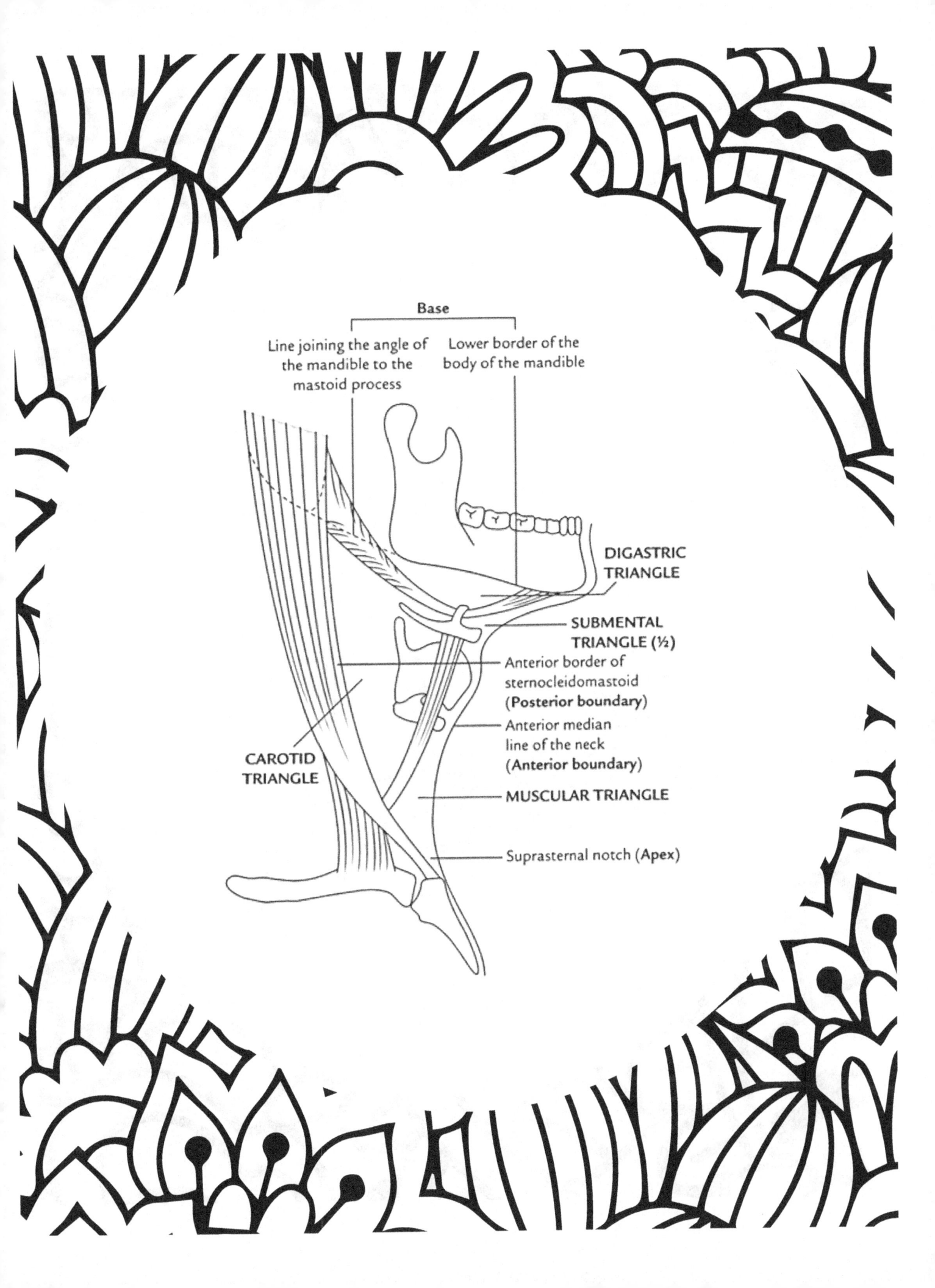

Line joining the angle of the mandible to the mastoid process | Lower border of the body of the mandible

DIGASTRIC TRIANGLE

SUBMENTAL TRIANGLE (½)

Anterior border of sternocleidomastoid (Posterior boundary)

Anterior median line of the neck (Anterior boundary)

CAROTID TRIANGLE

MUSCULAR TRIANGLE

Suprasternal notch (Apex)

Resistance

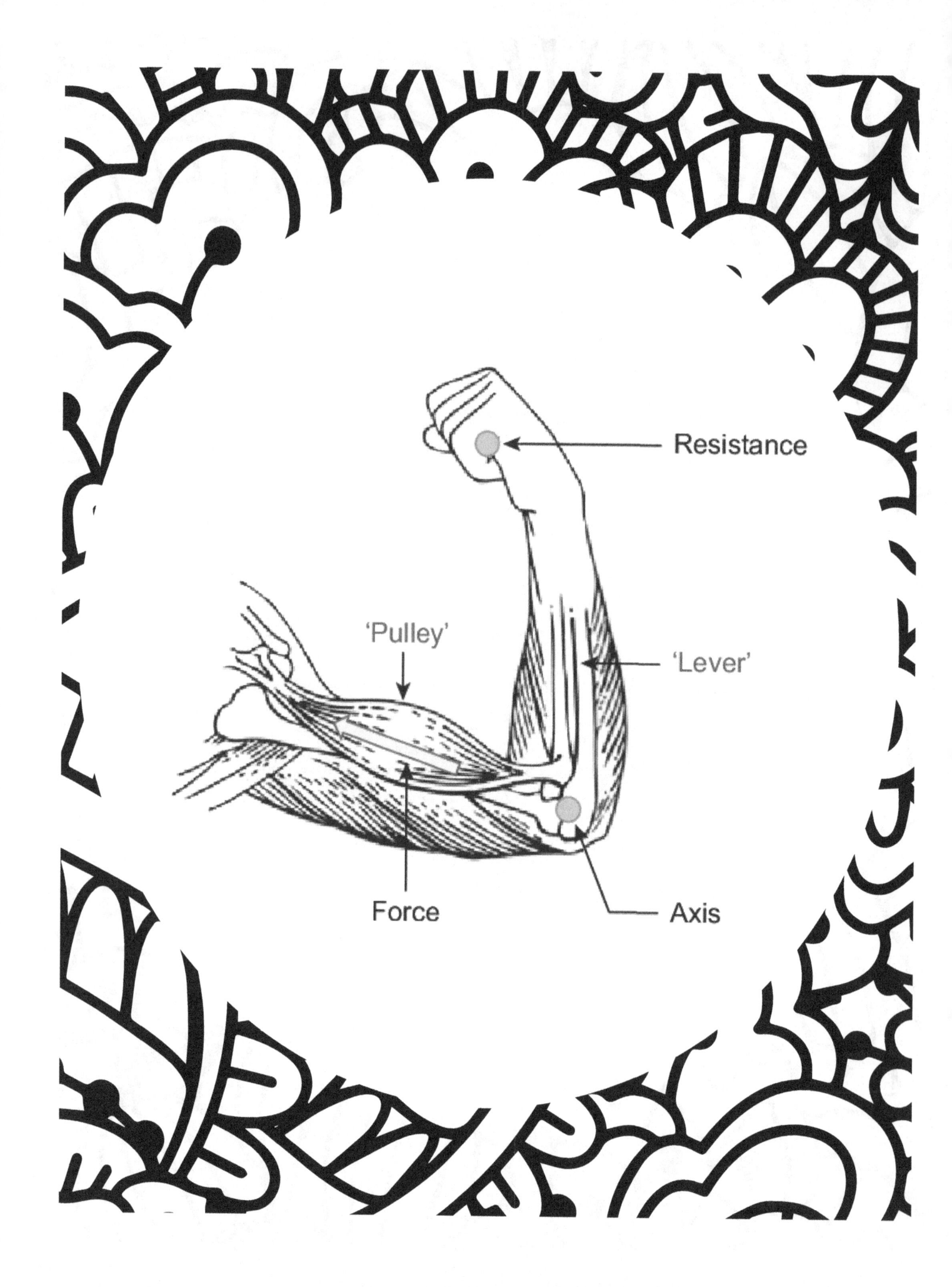

'Pulley'

'Lever'

Force

Axis

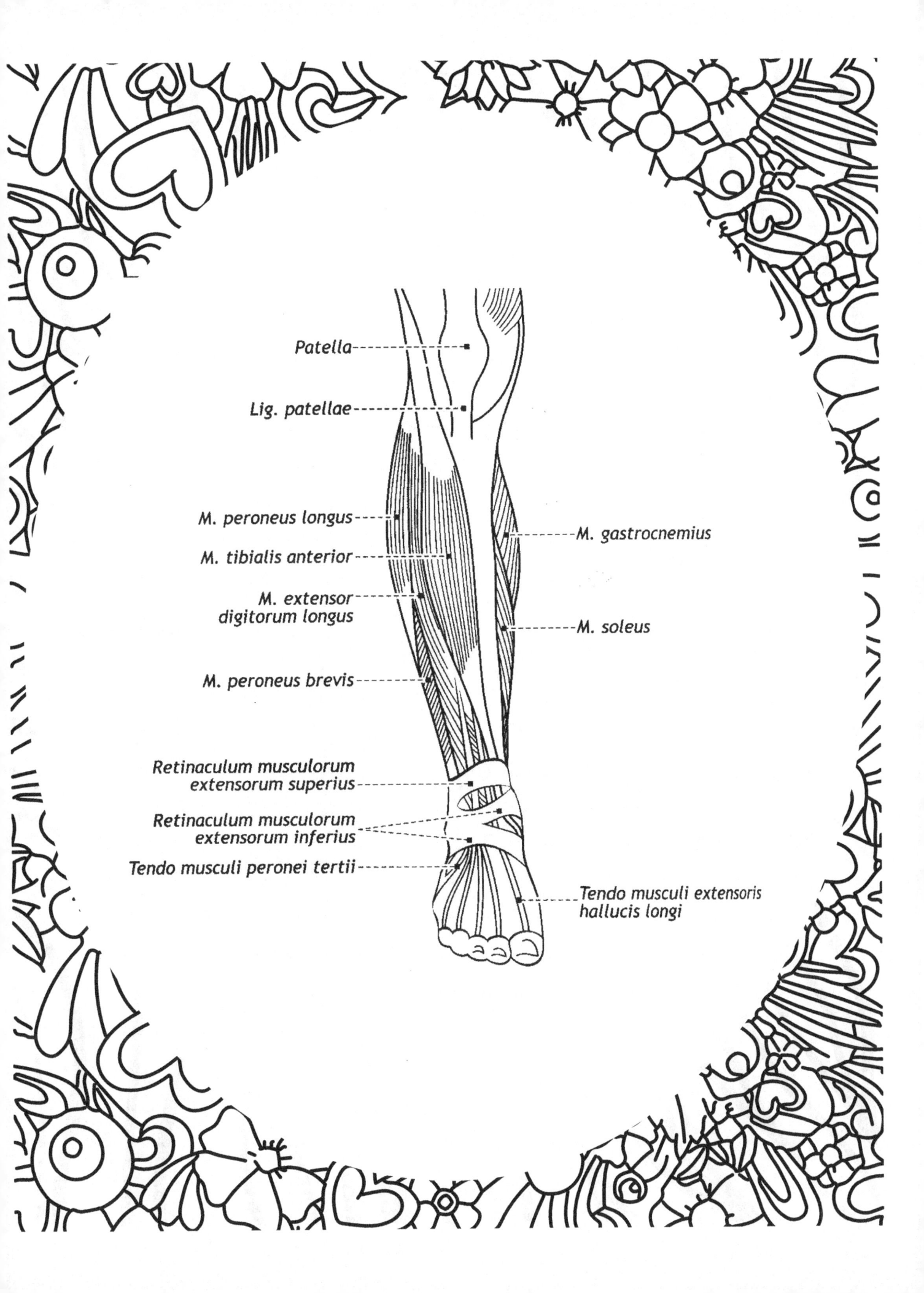

- Patella
- Lig. patellae
- M. peroneus longus
- M. tibialis anterior
- M. extensor digitorum longus
- M. peroneus brevis
- Retinaculum musculorum extensorum superius
- Retinaculum musculorum extensorum inferius
- Tendo musculi peronei tertii
- M. gastrocnemius
- M. soleus
- Tendo musculi extensoris hallucis longi

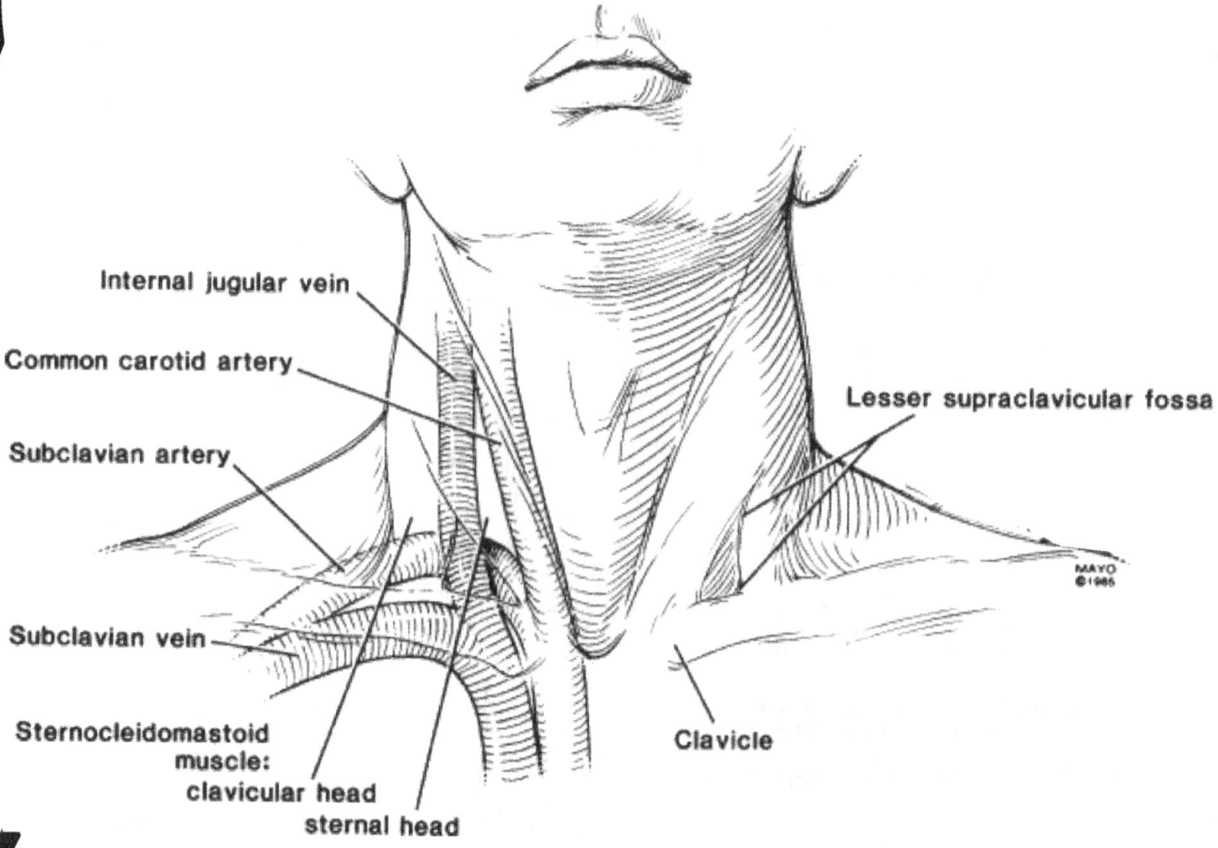

Internal jugular vein
Common carotid artery
Subclavian artery
Subclavian vein
Sternocleidomastoid
muscle:
clavicular head
sternal head
Lesser supraclavicular fossa
Clavicle
MAYO

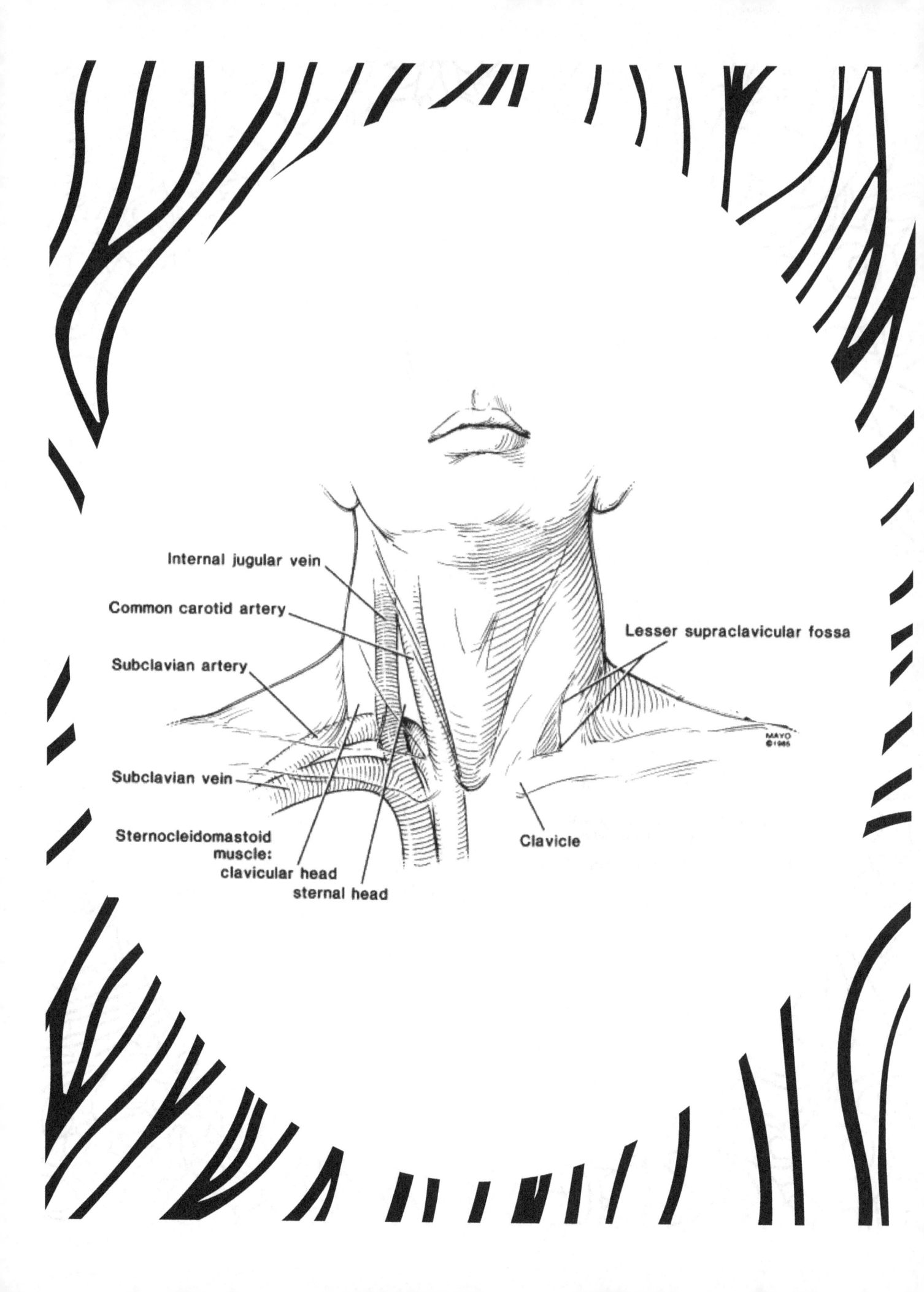

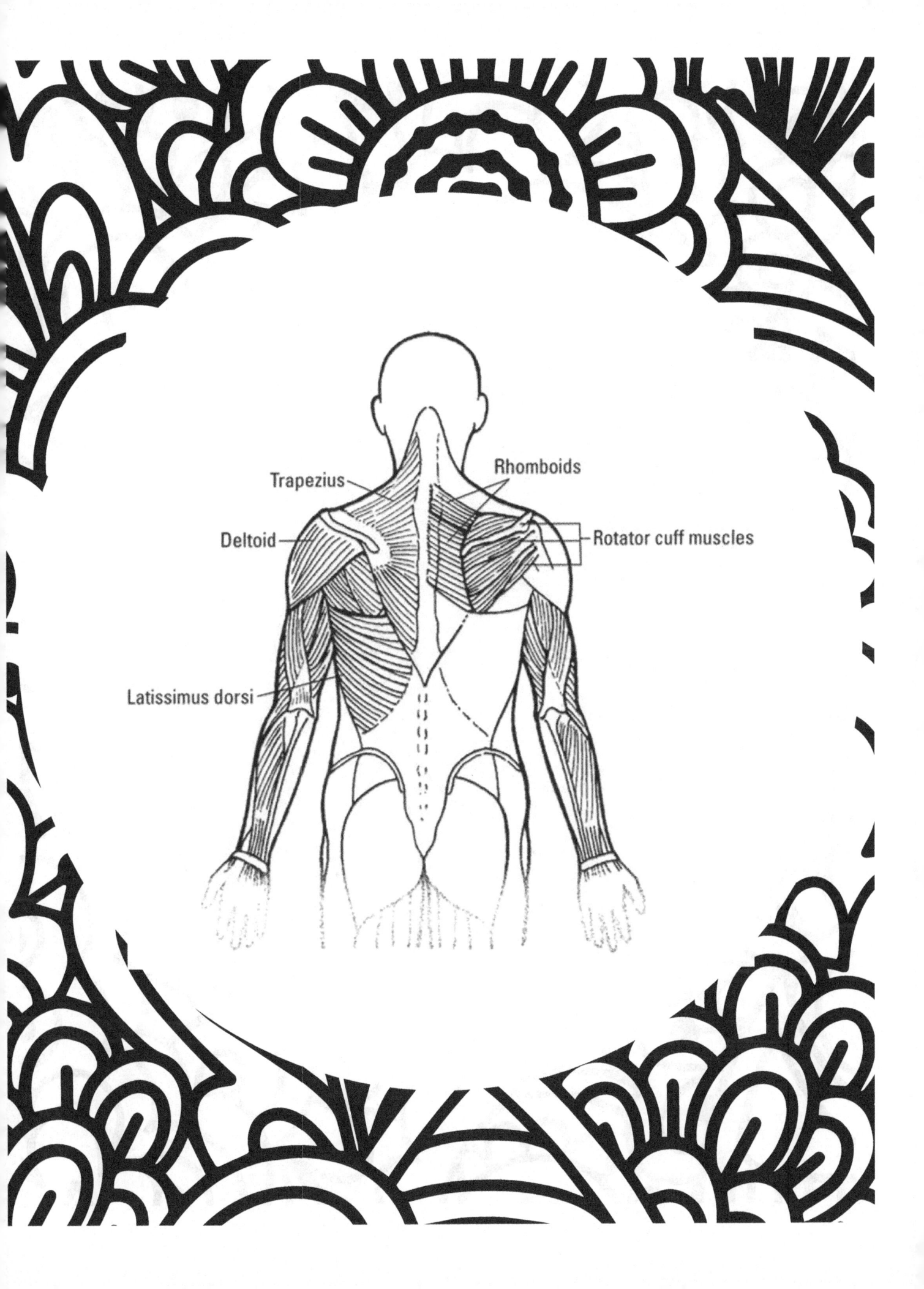

- Trapezius
- Rhomboids
- Deltoid
- Rotator cuff muscles
- Latissimus dorsi

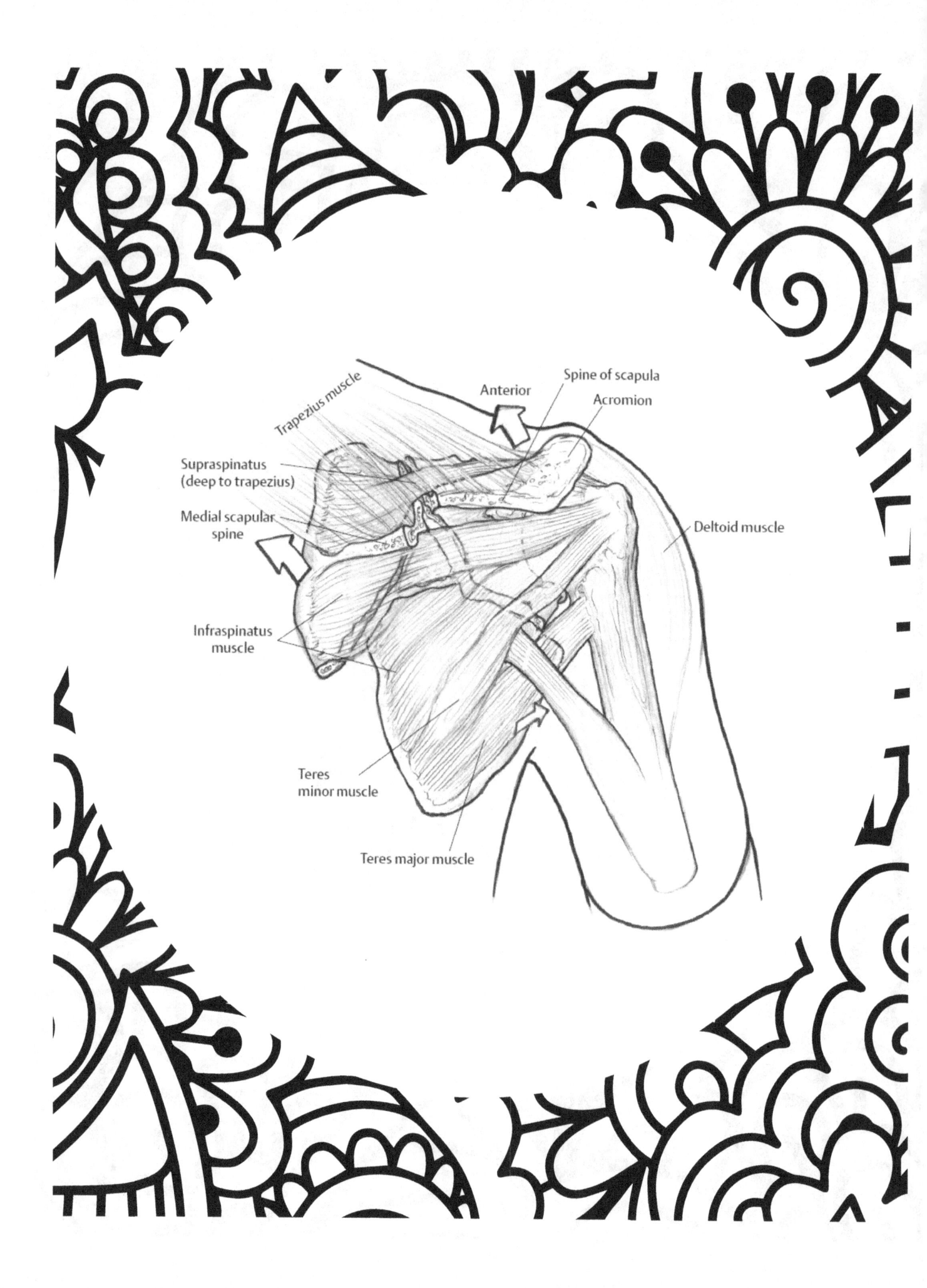

- Trapezius muscle
- Anterior
- Spine of scapula
- Acromion
- Supraspinatus (deep to trapezius)
- Medial scapular spine
- Deltoid muscle
- Infraspinatus muscle
- Teres minor muscle
- Teres major muscle

a

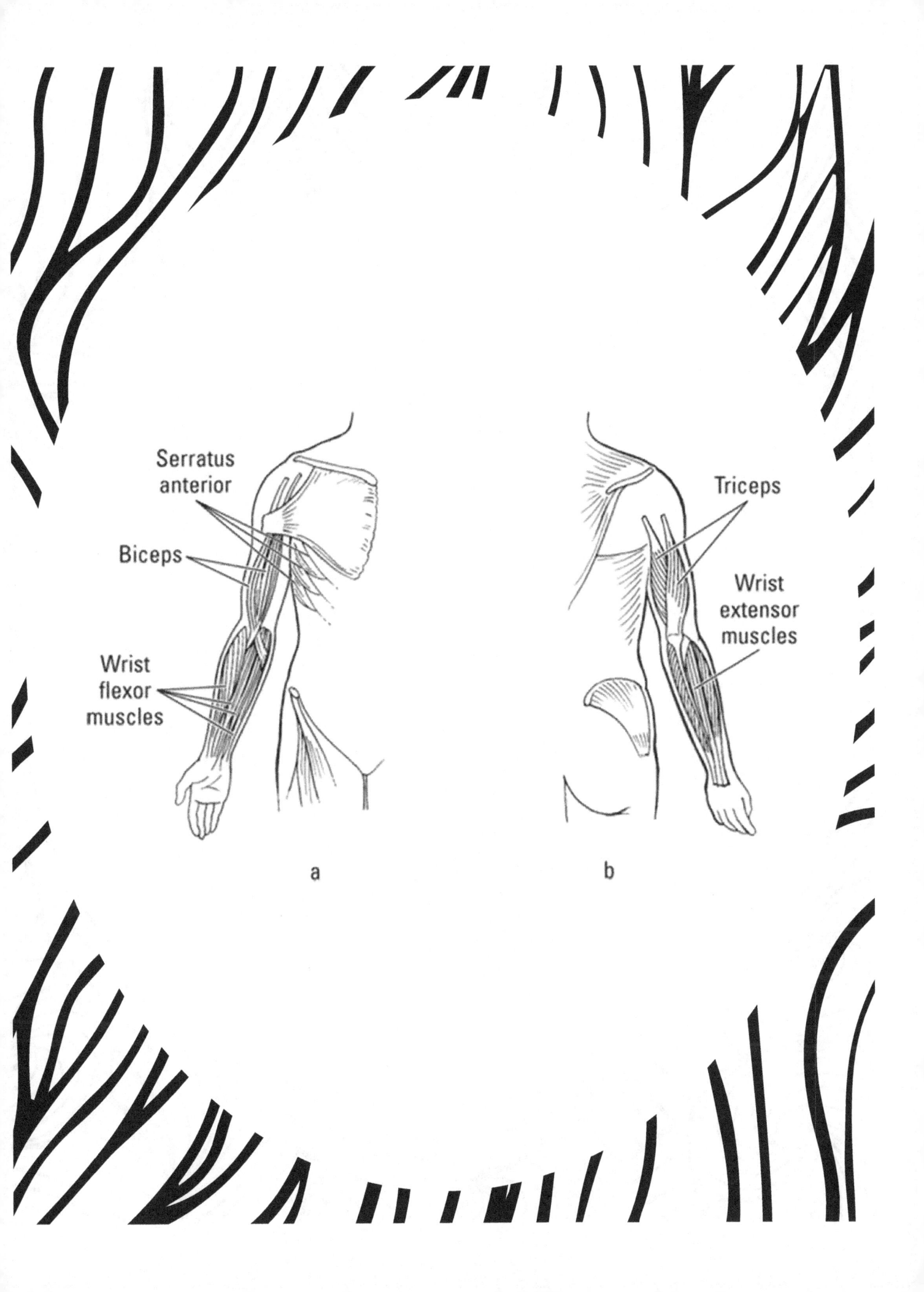

b

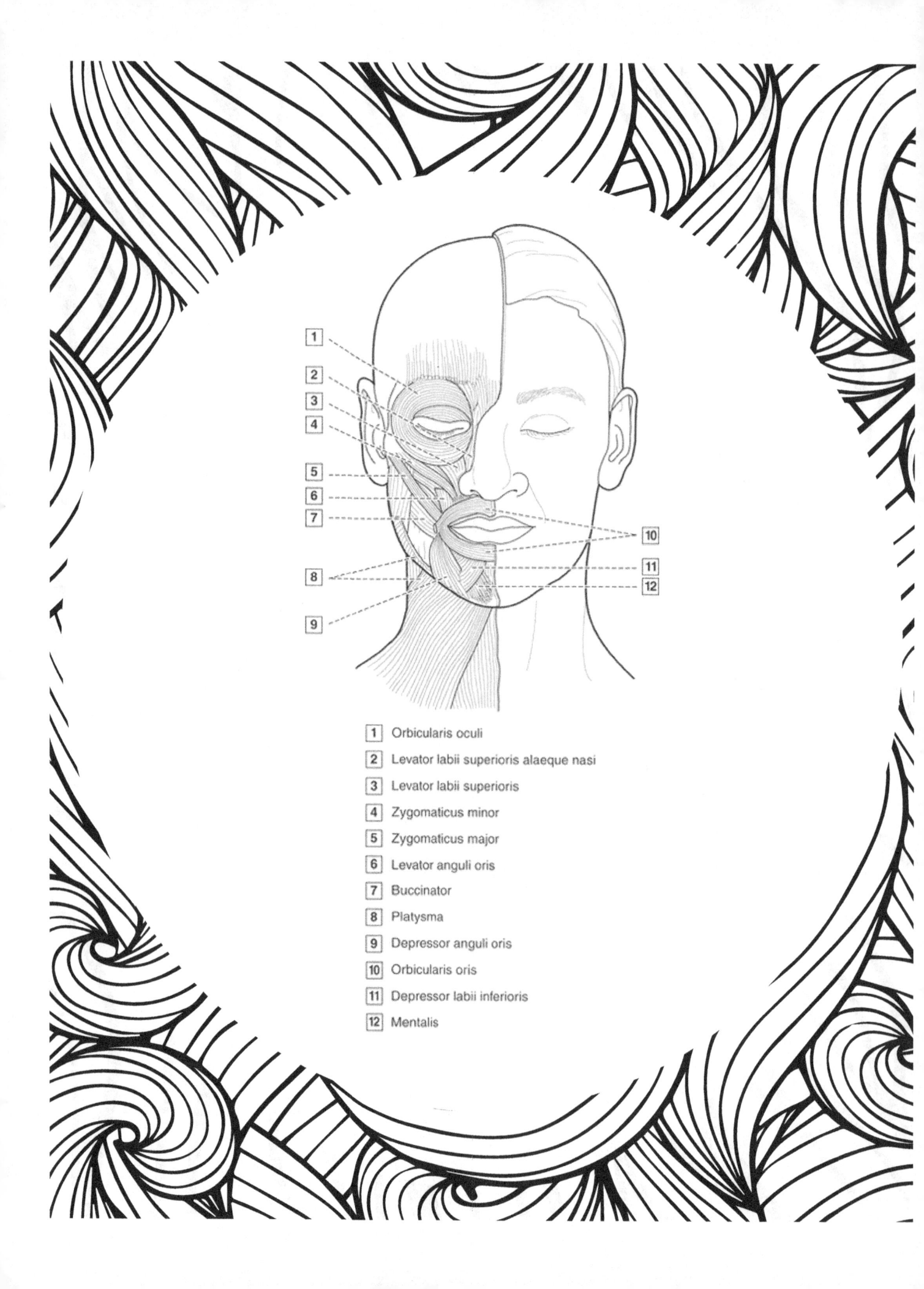

1 Orbicularis oculi
2 Levator labii superioris alaeque nasi
3 Levator labii superioris
4 Zygomaticus minor
5 Zygomaticus major
6 Levator anguli oris
7 Buccinator
8 Platysma
9 Depressor anguli oris
10 Orbicularis oris
11 Depressor labii inferioris
12 Mentalis

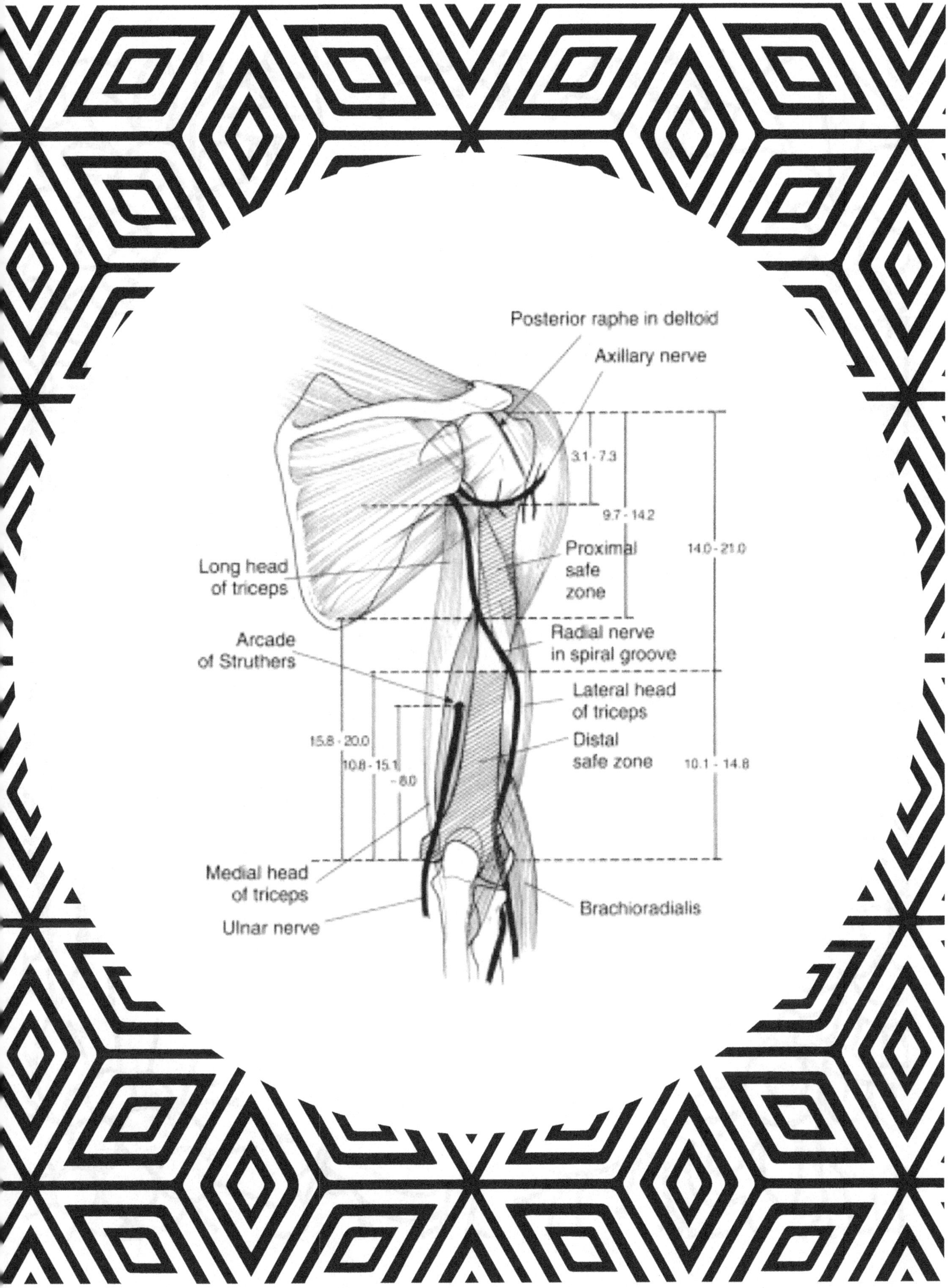
Posterior raphe in deltoid
Axillary nerve
3.1 - 7.3
9.7 - 14.2
14.0 - 21.0
Long head
of triceps
Proximal
safe
zone
Arcade
of Struthers
Radial nerve
in spiral groove
Lateral head
of triceps
15.8 - 20.0
10.8 - 15.1
- 8.0
Distal
safe zone
10.1 - 14.8
Medial head
of triceps
Ulnar nerve
Brachioradialis

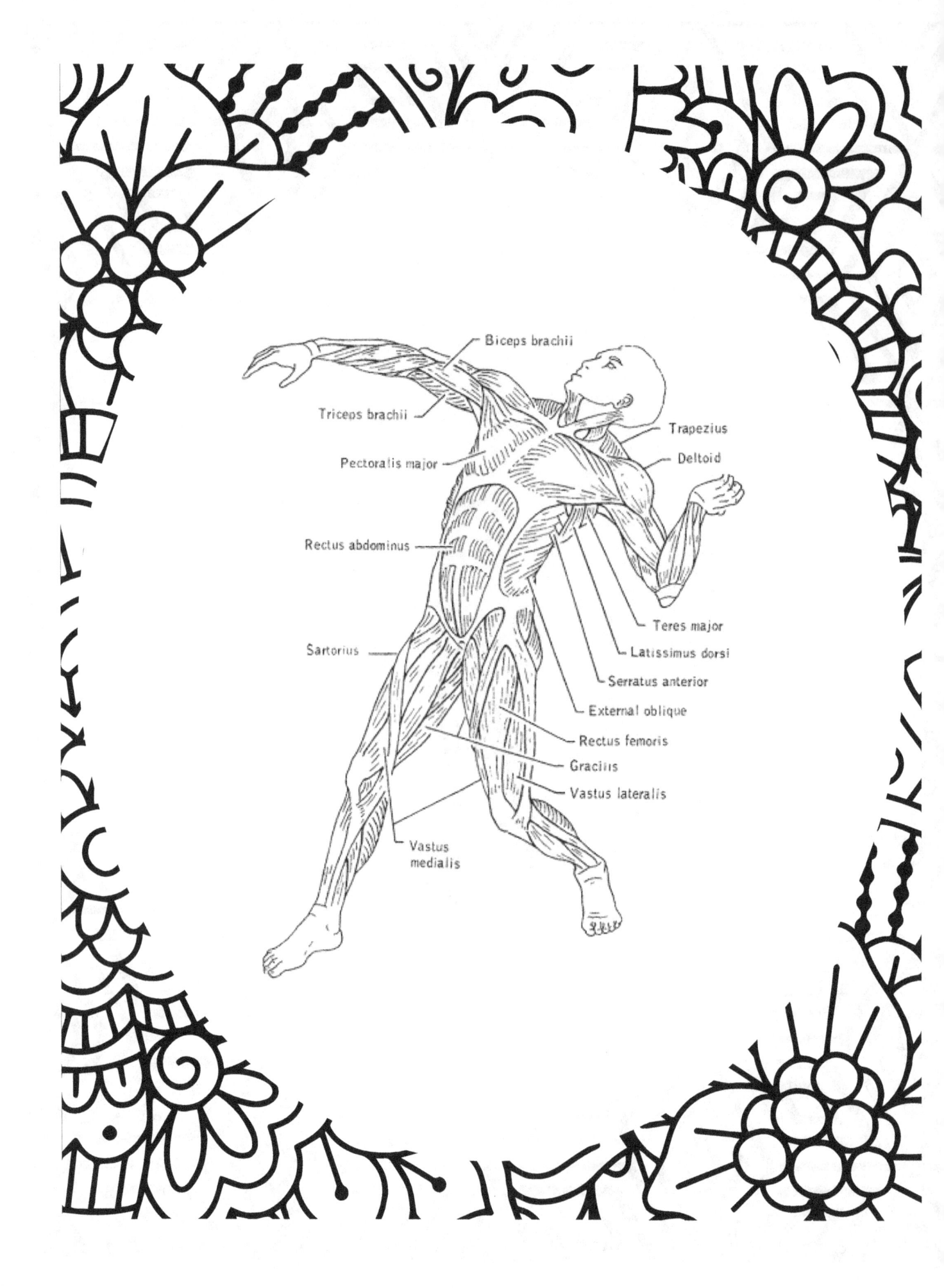

- Biceps brachii
- Triceps brachii
- Trapezius
- Pectoralis major
- Deltoid
- Rectus abdominus
- Sartorius
- Teres major
- Latissimus dorsi
- Serratus anterior
- External oblique
- Rectus femoris
- Gracilis
- Vastus lateralis
- Vastus medialis

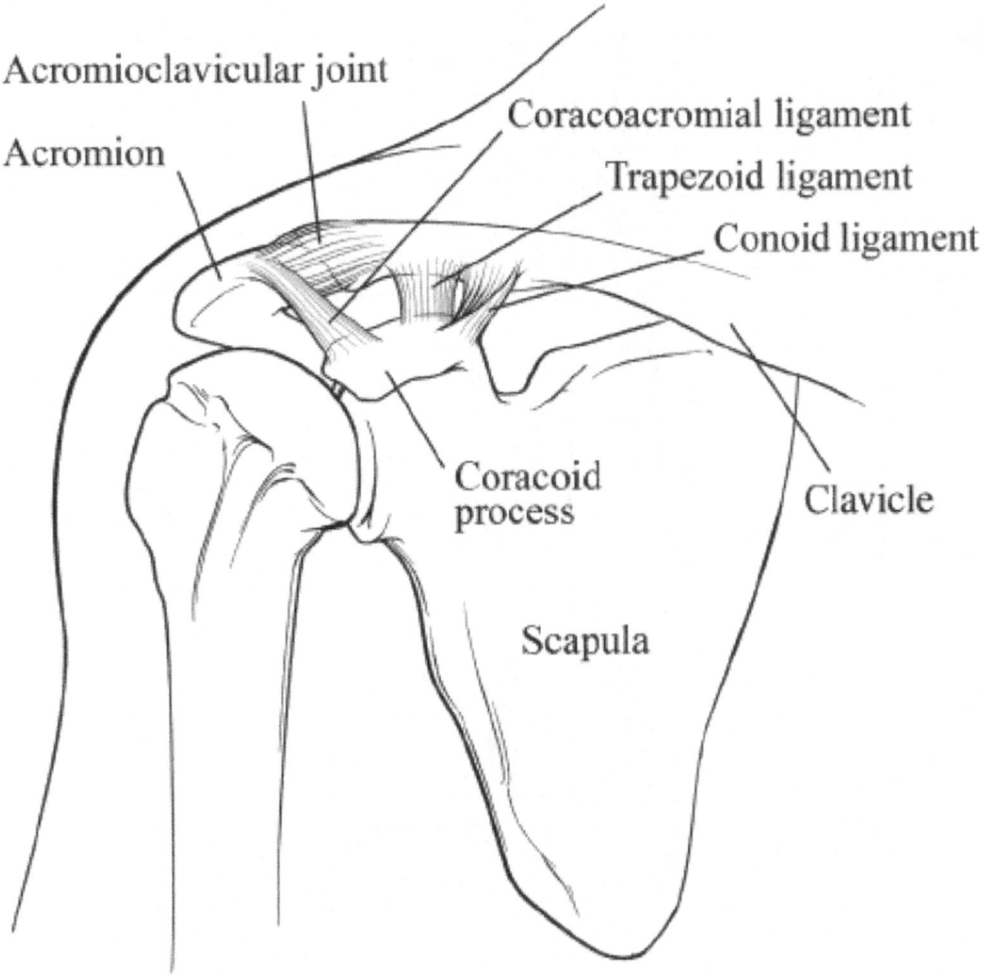

Acromioclavicular joint
Coracoacromial ligament
Acromion
Trapezoid ligament
Conoid ligament
Coracoid process
Clavicle
Scapula

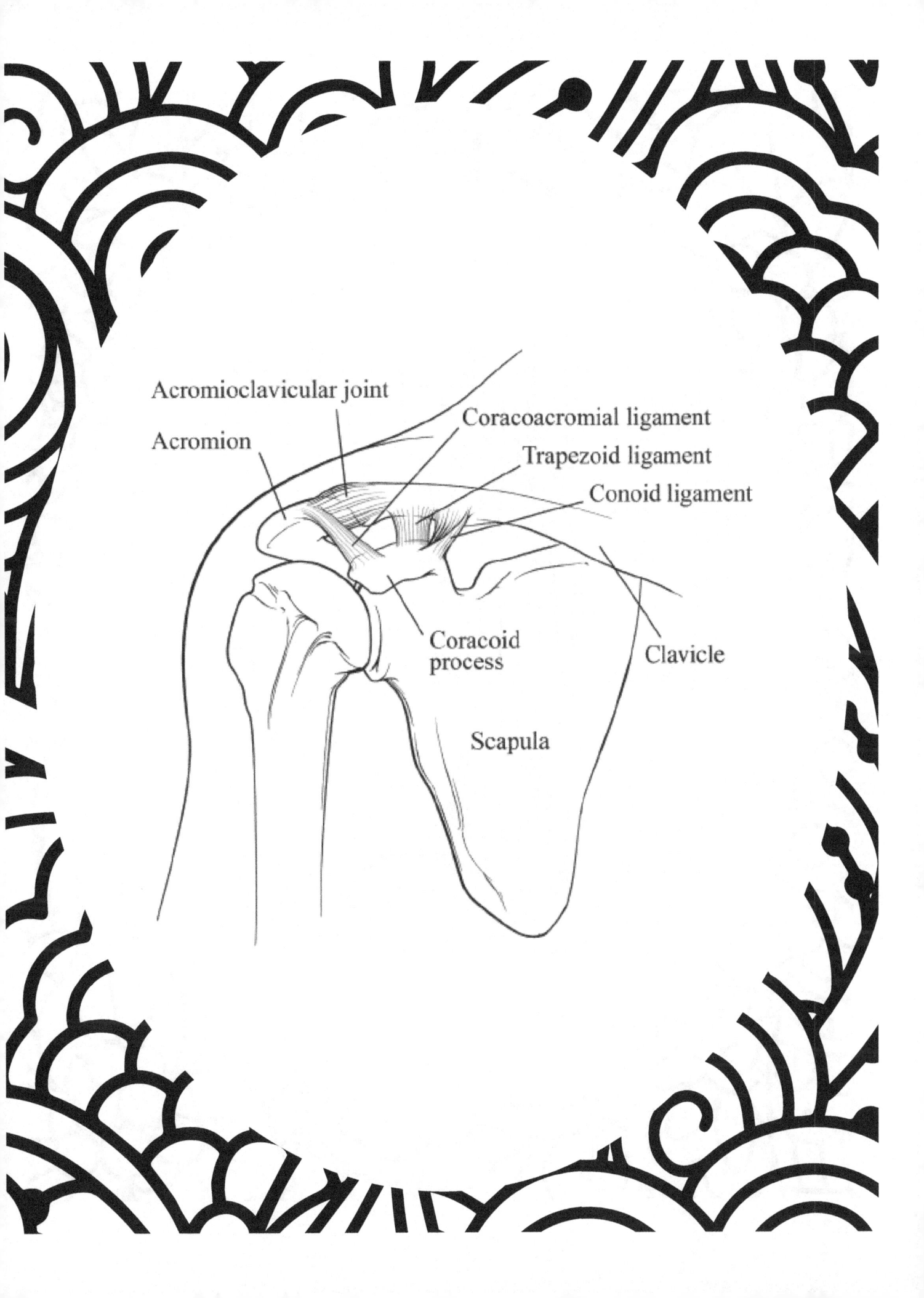

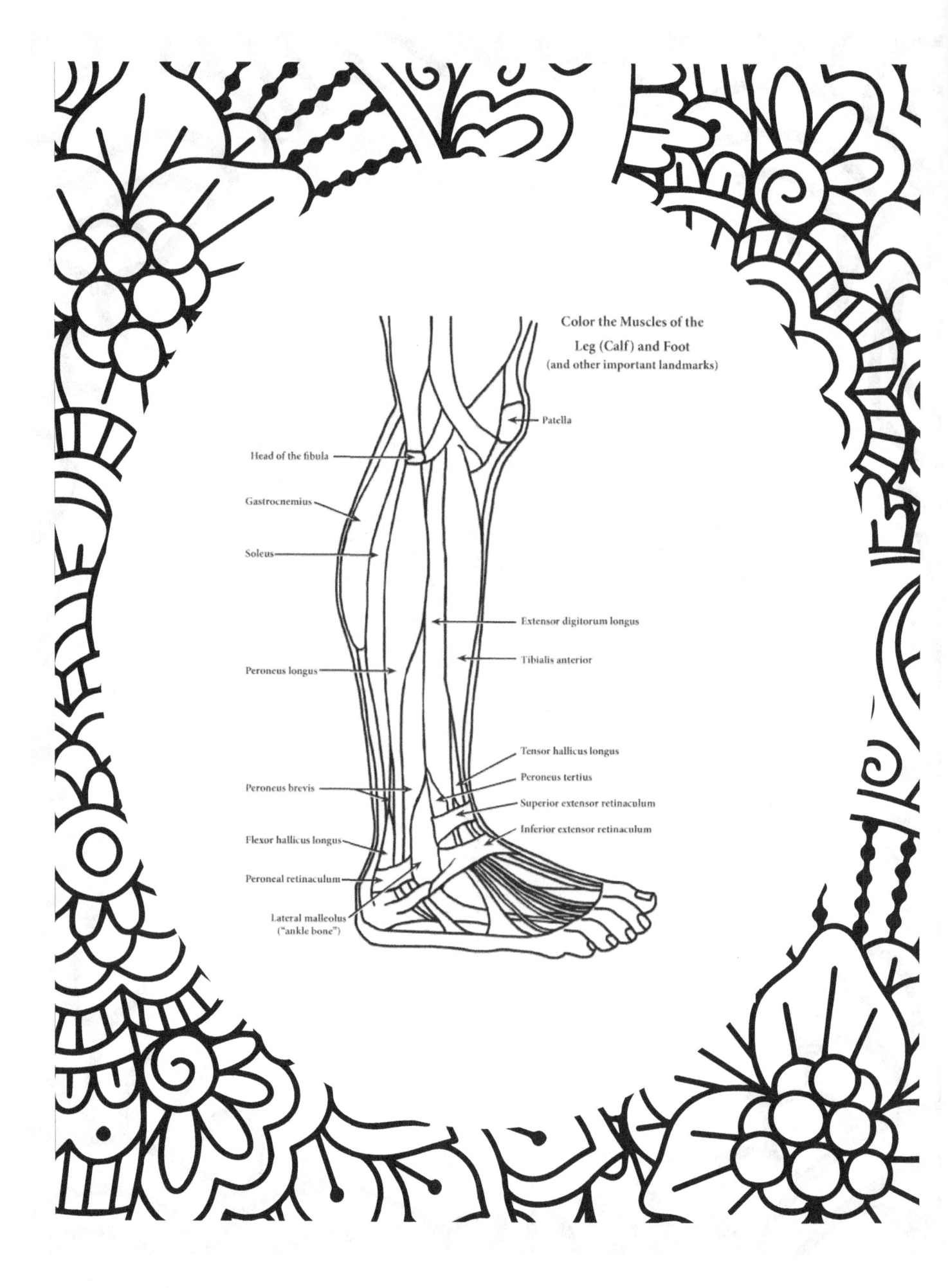

**Color the Muscles of the
Leg (Calf) and Foot**
(and other important landmarks)

- Patella
- Head of the fibula
- Gastrocnemius
- Soleus
- Extensor digitorum longus
- Tibialis anterior
- Peroneus longus
- Tensor hallicus longus
- Peroneus tertius
- Superior extensor retinaculum
- Peroneus brevis
- Inferior extensor retinaculum
- Flexor hallicus longus
- Peroneal retinaculum
- Lateral malleolus ("ankle bone")

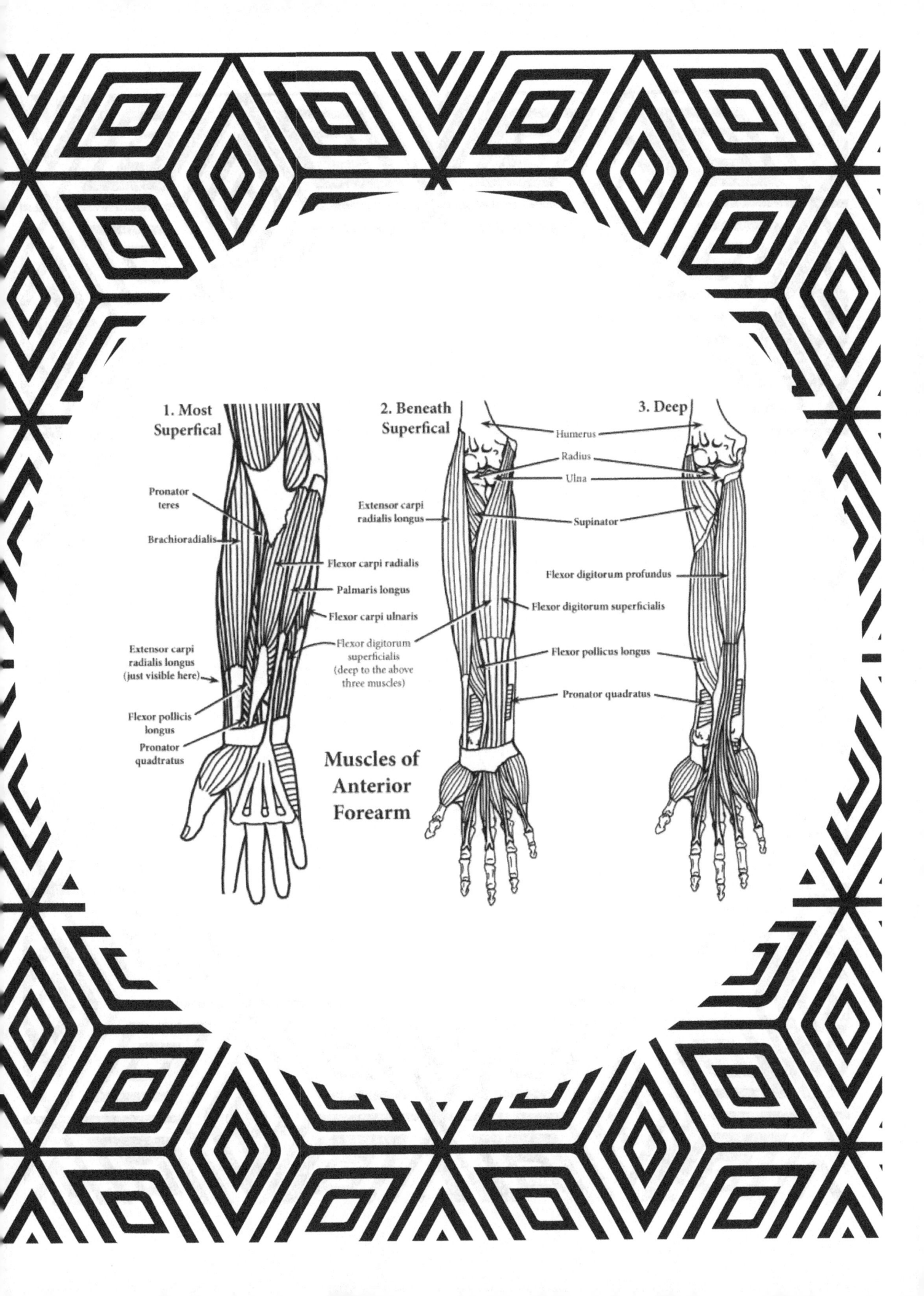

1. Most Superfical
- Pronator teres
- Brachioradialis
- Flexor carpi radialis
- Palmaris longus
- Flexor carpi ulnaris
- Extensor carpi radialis longus (just visible here)
- Flexor digitorum superficialis (deep to the above three muscles)
- Flexor pollicis longus
- Pronator quadratus

2. Beneath Superfical
- Extensor carpi radialis longus
- Flexor digitorum superficialis

3. Deep
- Humerus
- Radius
- Ulna
- Supinator
- Flexor digitorum profundus
- Flexor pollicus longus
- Pronator quadratus

Muscles of Anterior Forearm

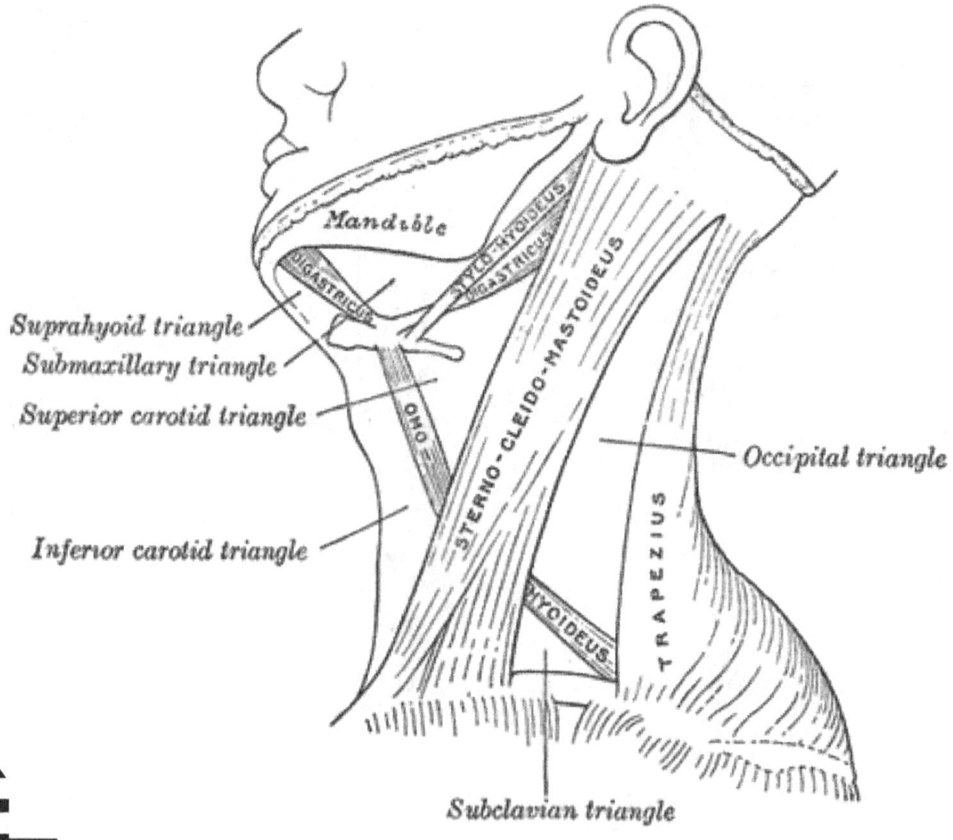
Mandible
DIGASTRICUS
STYLO-HYOIDEUS
DIGASTRICUS
Suprahyoid triangle
Submaxillary triangle
Superior carotid triangle
OMO
STERNO-CLEIDO-MASTOIDEUS
Occipital triangle
TRAPEZIUS
Inferior carotid triangle
HYOIDEUS
Subclavian triangle

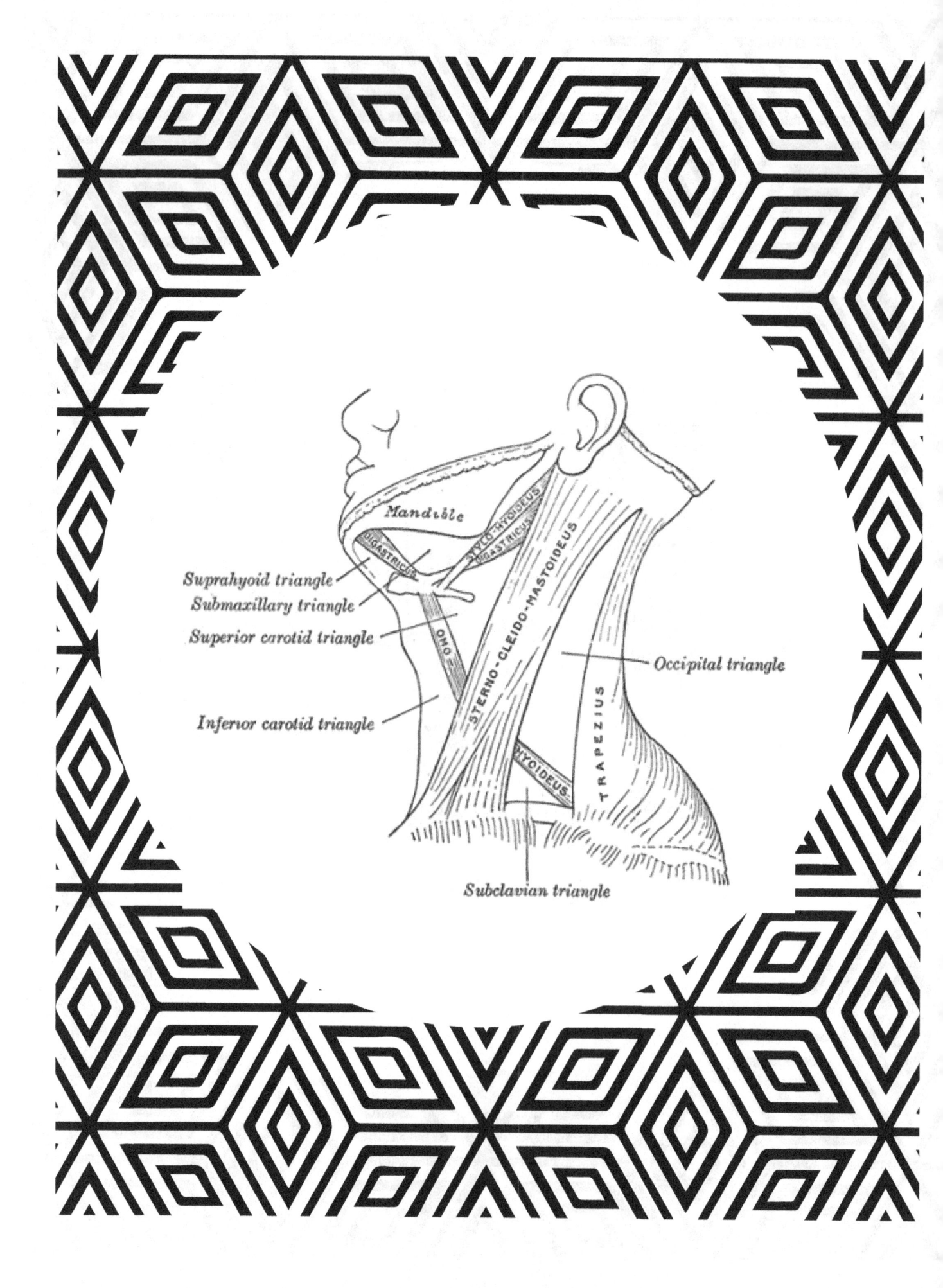

PROXIMAL

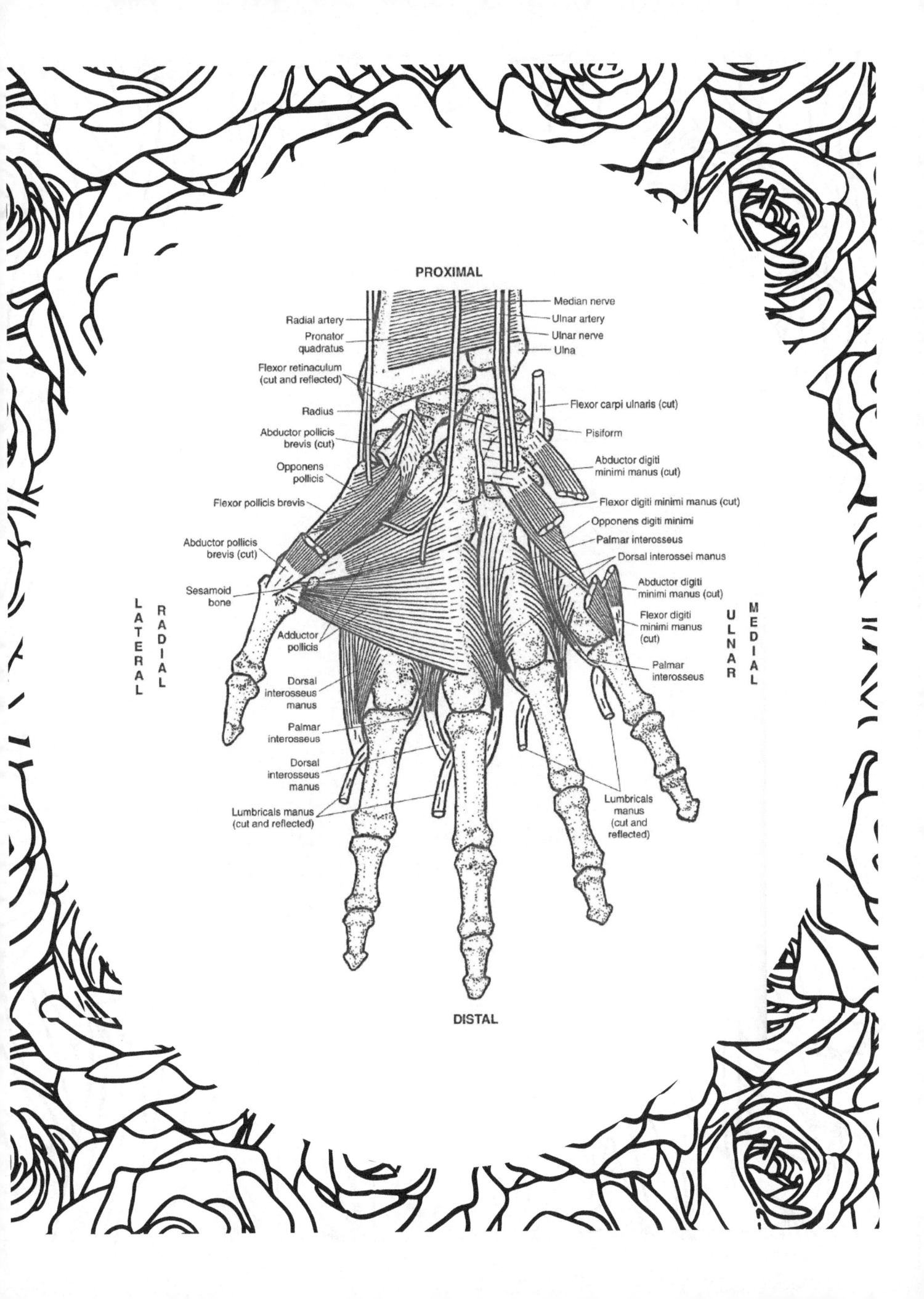

- Radial artery
- Pronator quadratus
- Flexor retinaculum (cut and reflected)
- Radius
- Abductor pollicis brevis (cut)
- Opponens pollicis
- Flexor pollicis brevis
- Abductor pollicis brevis (cut)
- Sesamoid bone
- Adductor pollicis
- Dorsal interosseus manus
- Palmar interosseus
- Dorsal interosseus manus
- Lumbricals manus (cut and reflected)

- Median nerve
- Ulnar artery
- Ulnar nerve
- Ulna
- Flexor carpi ulnaris (cut)
- Pisiform
- Abductor digiti minimi manus (cut)
- Flexor digiti minimi manus (cut)
- Opponens digiti minimi
- Palmar interosseus
- Dorsal interossei manus
- Abductor digiti minimi manus (cut)
- Flexor digiti minimi manus (cut)
- Palmar interosseus
- Lumbricals manus (cut and reflected)

LATERAL RADIAL   **ULNAR MEDIAL**

DISTAL

Anterior

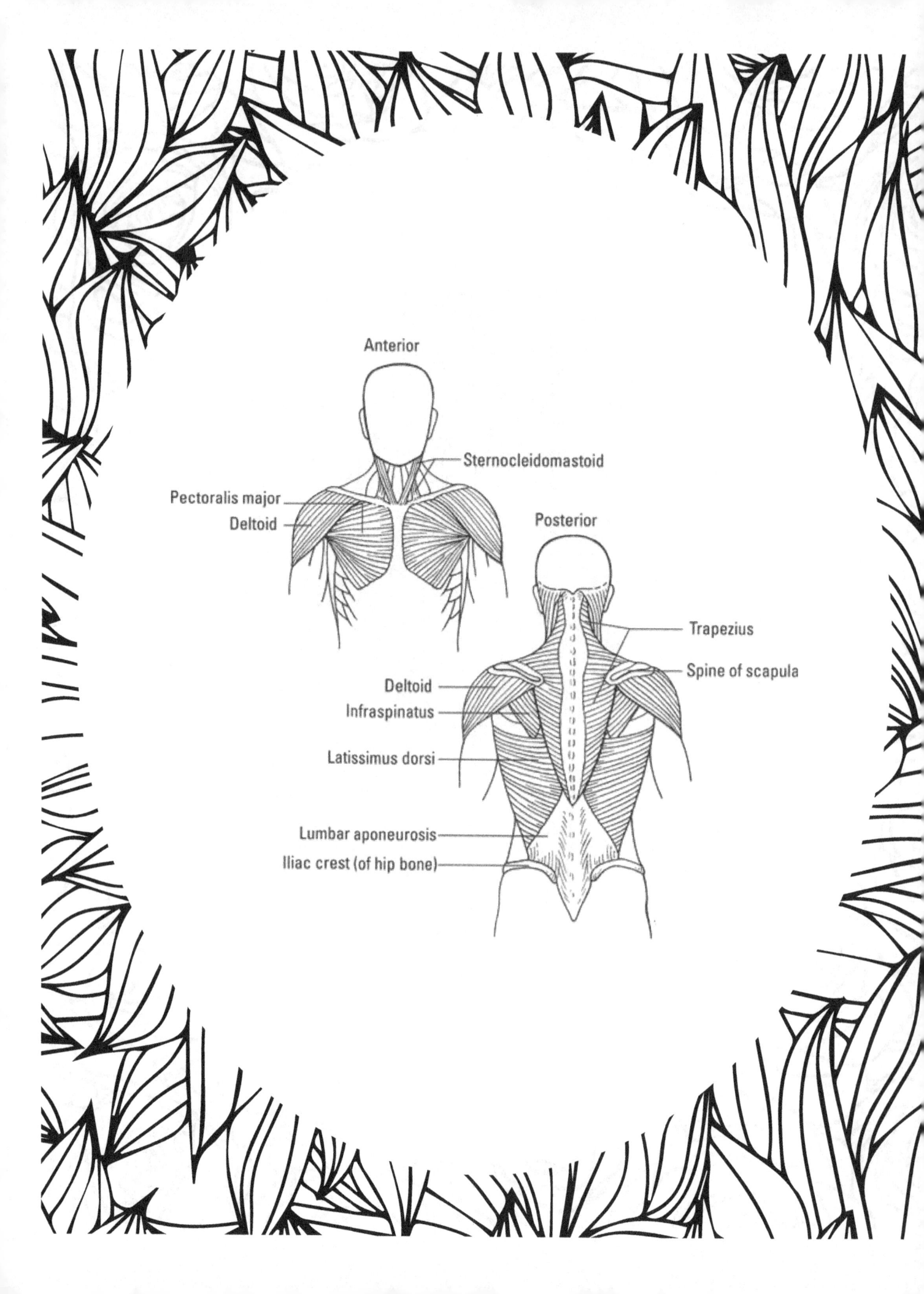

- Sternocleidomastoid
- Pectoralis major
- Deltoid

Posterior

- Trapezius
- Spine of scapula
- Deltoid
- Infraspinatus
- Latissimus dorsi
- Lumbar aponeurosis
- Iliac crest (of hip bone)

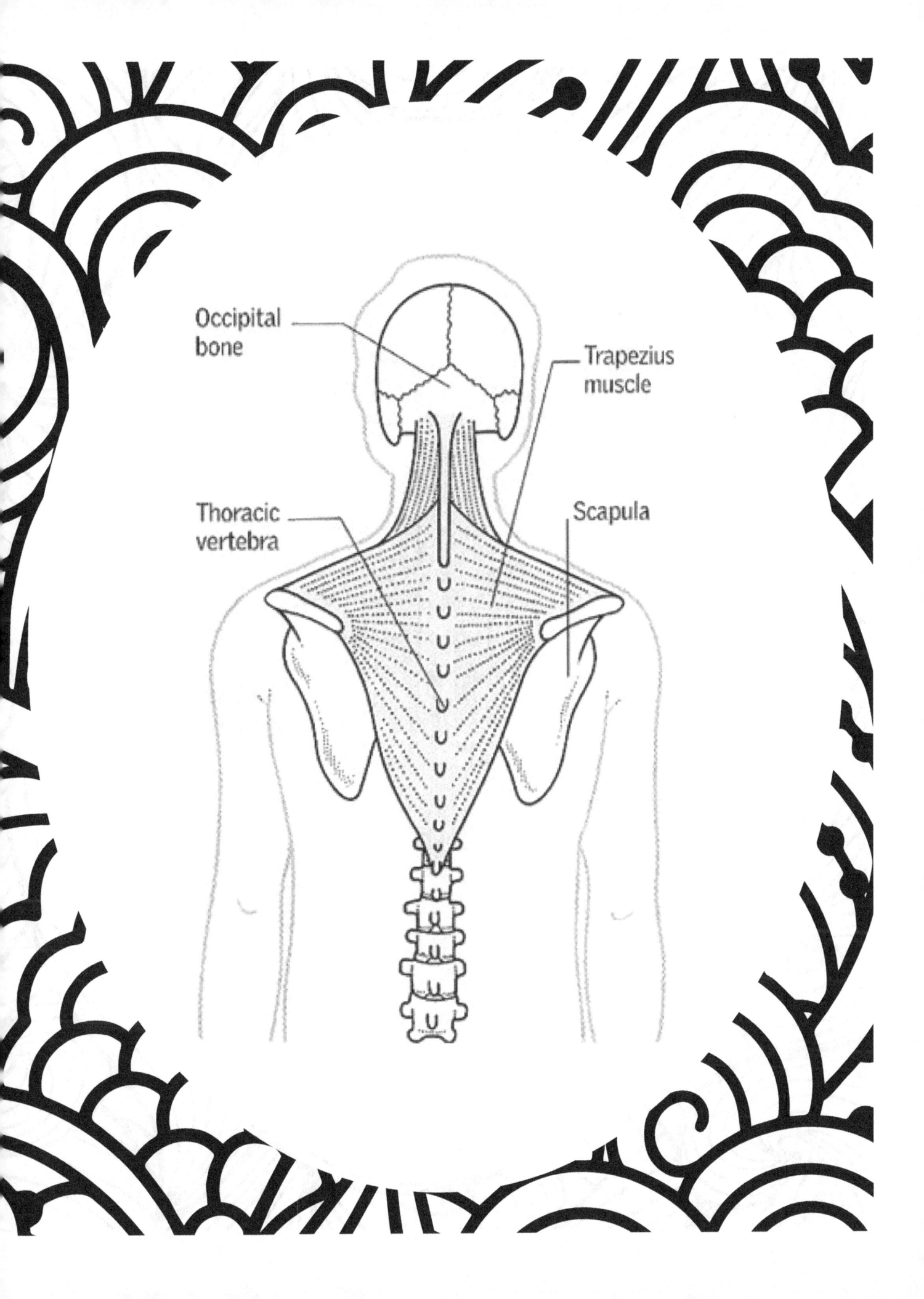

- Occipital bone
- Trapezius muscle
- Thoracic vertebra
- Scapula

(X-U)/2

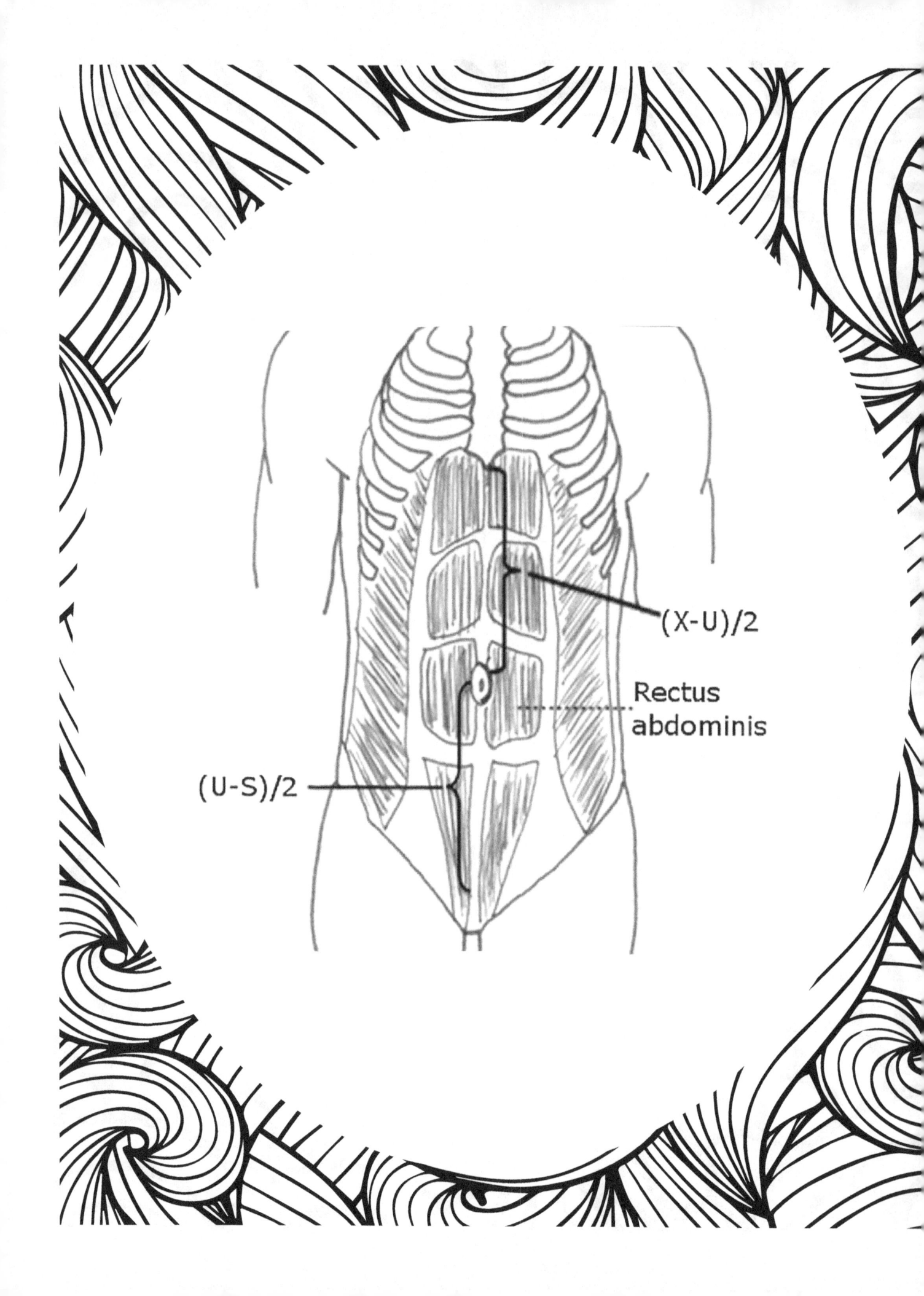

Rectus abdominis

(U-S)/2

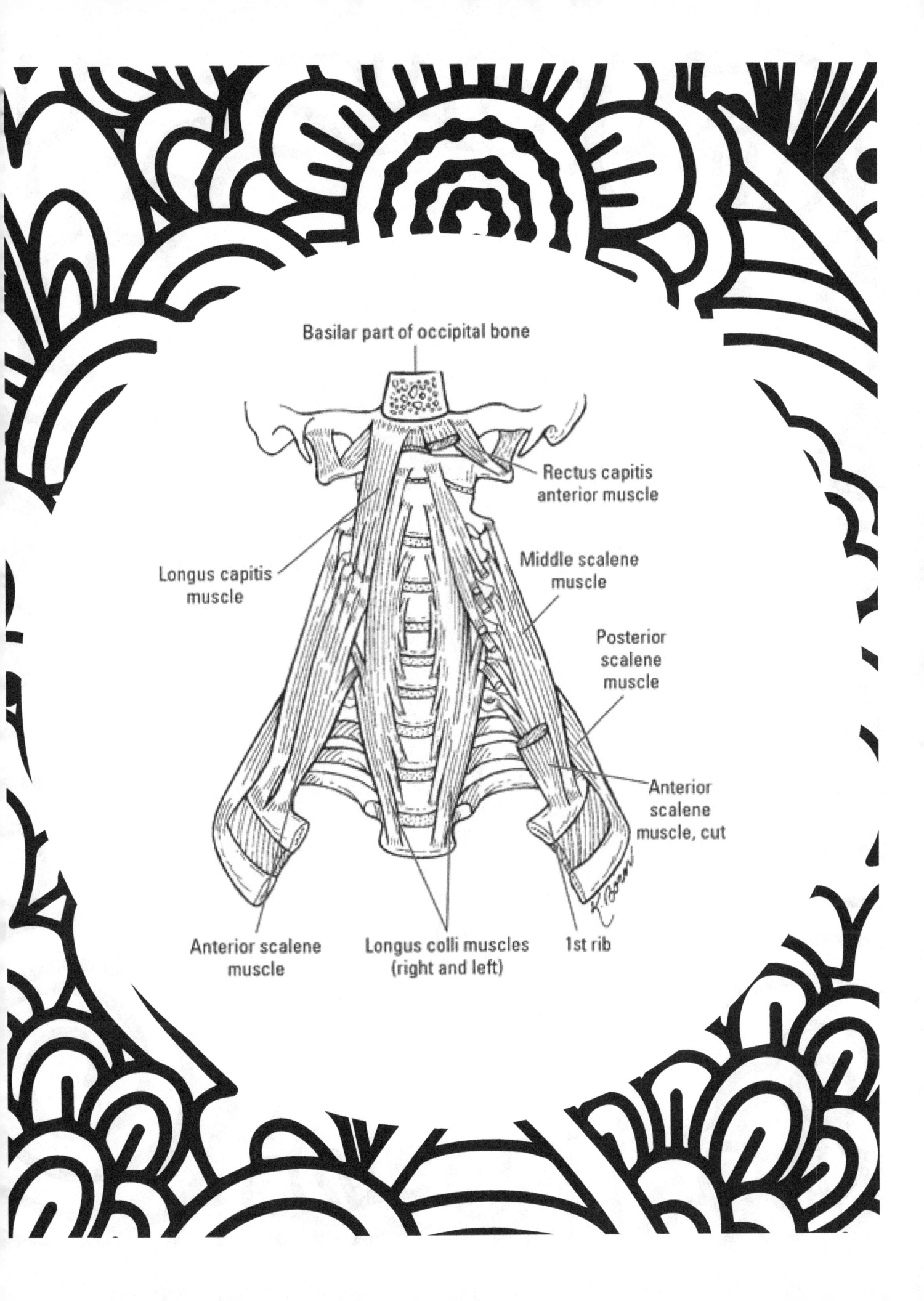

- Basilar part of occipital bone
- Rectus capitis anterior muscle
- Longus capitis muscle
- Middle scalene muscle
- Posterior scalene muscle
- Anterior scalene muscle, cut
- Anterior scalene muscle
- Longus colli muscles (right and left)
- 1st rib

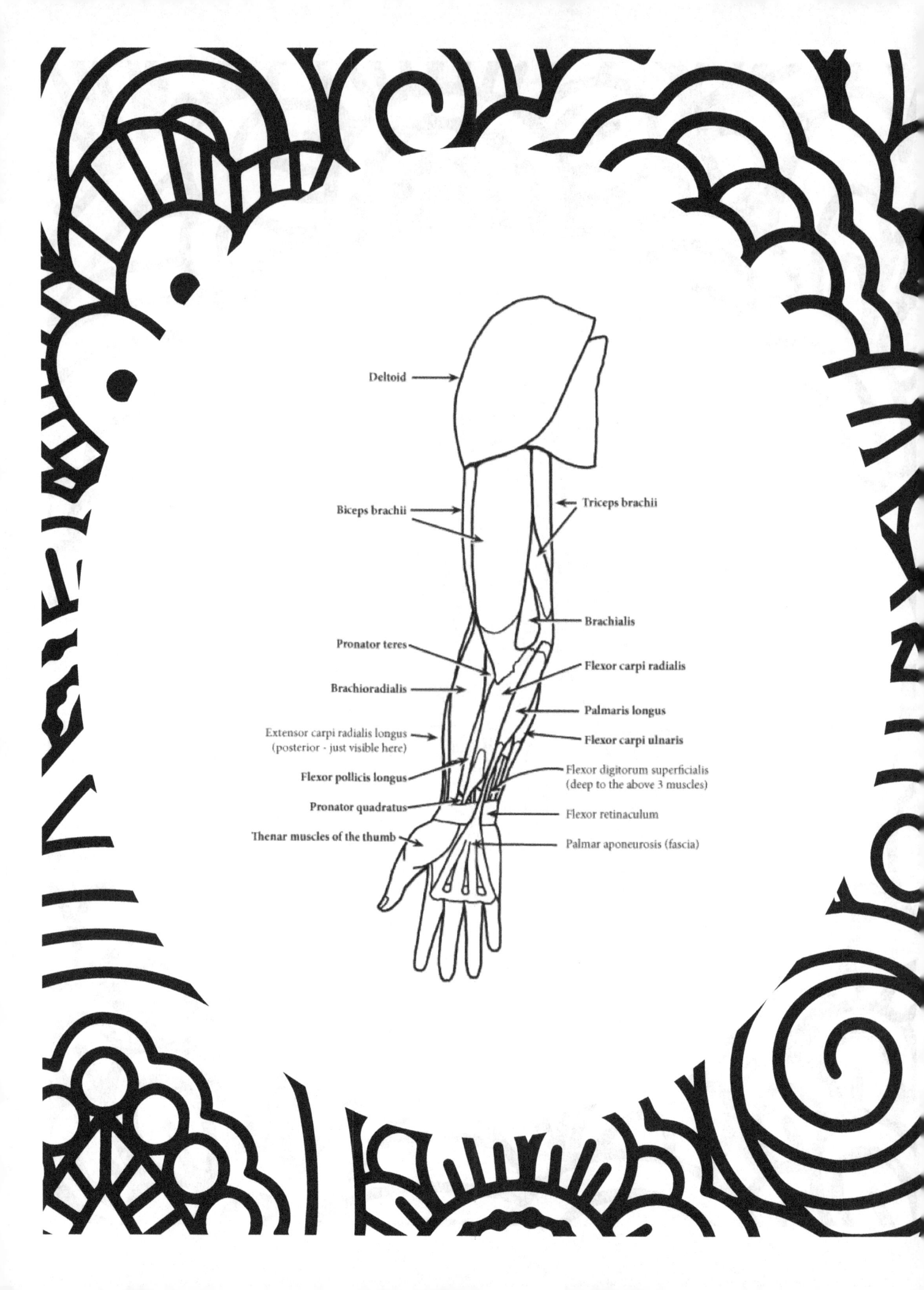

- Deltoid
- Biceps brachii
- Triceps brachii
- Brachialis
- Pronator teres
- Flexor carpi radialis
- Brachioradialis
- Palmaris longus
- Extensor carpi radialis longus (posterior - just visible here)
- Flexor carpi ulnaris
- Flexor pollicis longus
- Flexor digitorum superficialis (deep to the above 3 muscles)
- Pronator quadratus
- Flexor retinaculum
- Thenar muscles of the thumb
- Palmar aponeurosis (fascia)

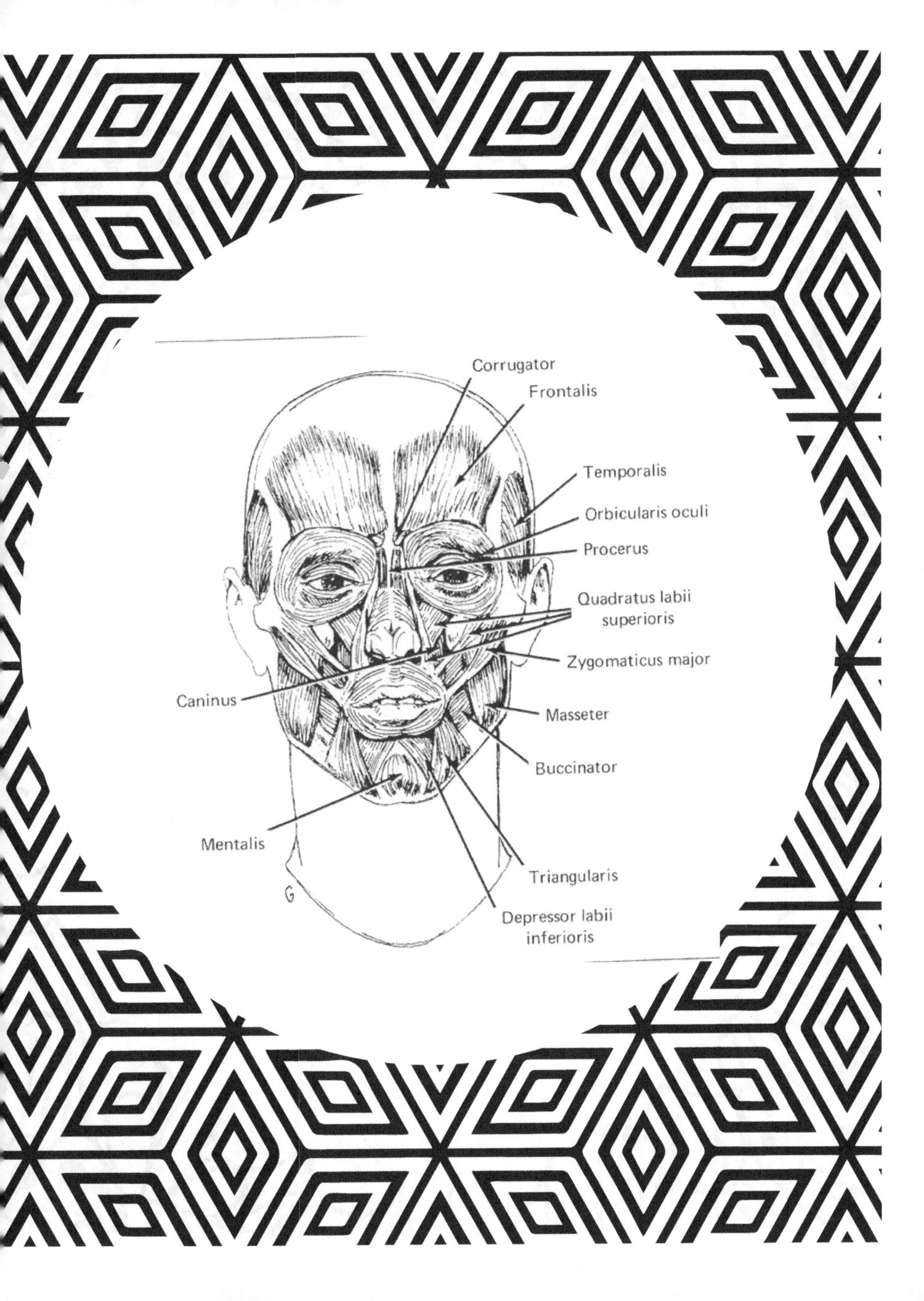

- Corrugator
- Frontalis
- Temporalis
- Orbicularis oculi
- Procerus
- Quadratus labii superioris
- Zygomaticus major
- Caninus
- Masseter
- Buccinator
- Mentalis
- Triangularis
- Depressor labii inferioris

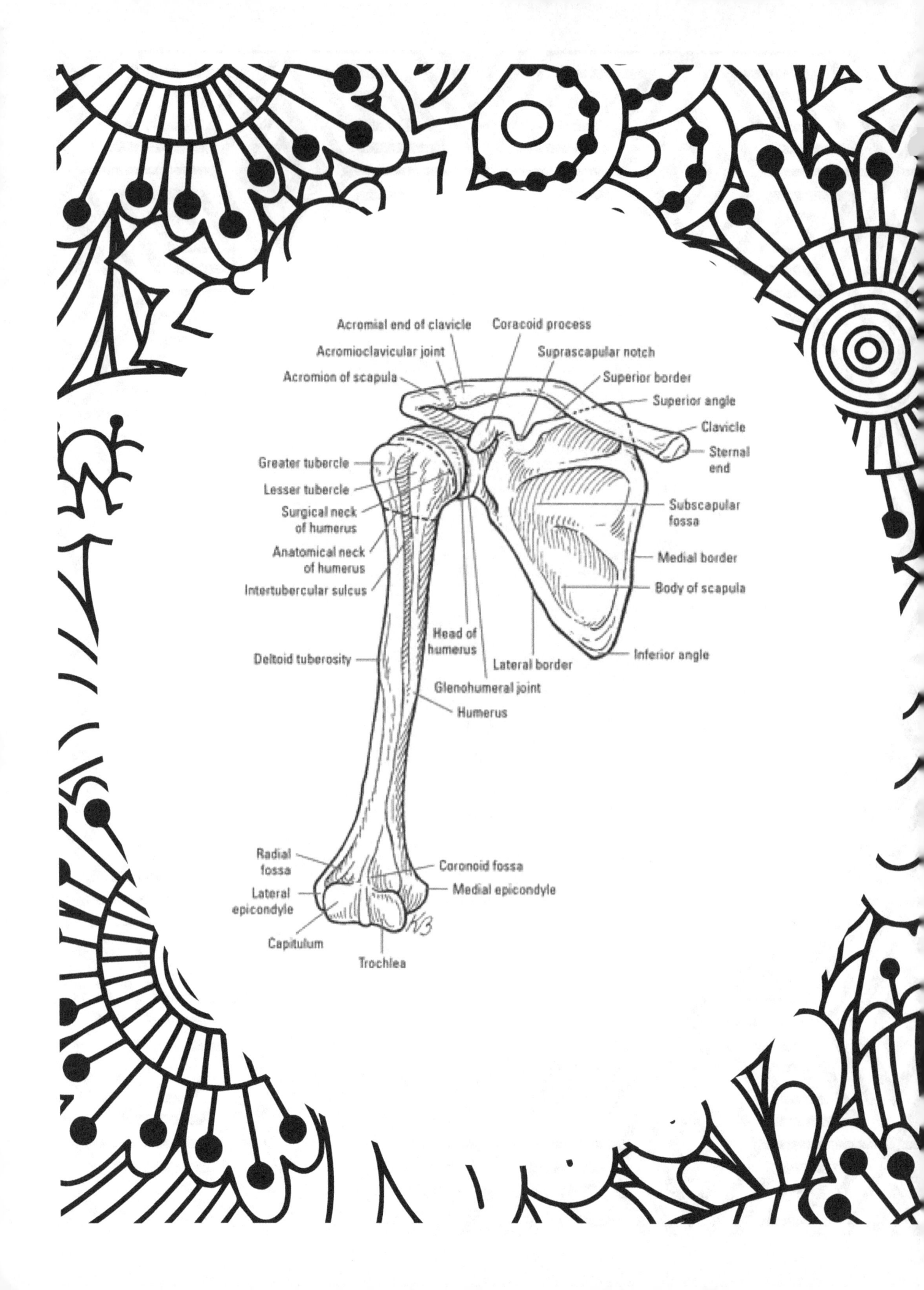

Acromial end of clavicle
Acromioclavicular joint
Acromion of scapula
Coracoid process
Suprascapular notch
Superior border
Superior angle
Clavicle
Sternal end
Greater tubercle
Lesser tubercle
Surgical neck of humerus
Anatomical neck of humerus
Intertubercular sulcus
Subscapular fossa
Medial border
Body of scapula
Head of humerus
Lateral border
Inferior angle
Deltoid tuberosity
Glenohumeral joint
Humerus
Radial fossa
Coronoid fossa
Medial epicondyle
Lateral epicondyle
Capitulum
Trochlea

ORBICULARIS OCULI

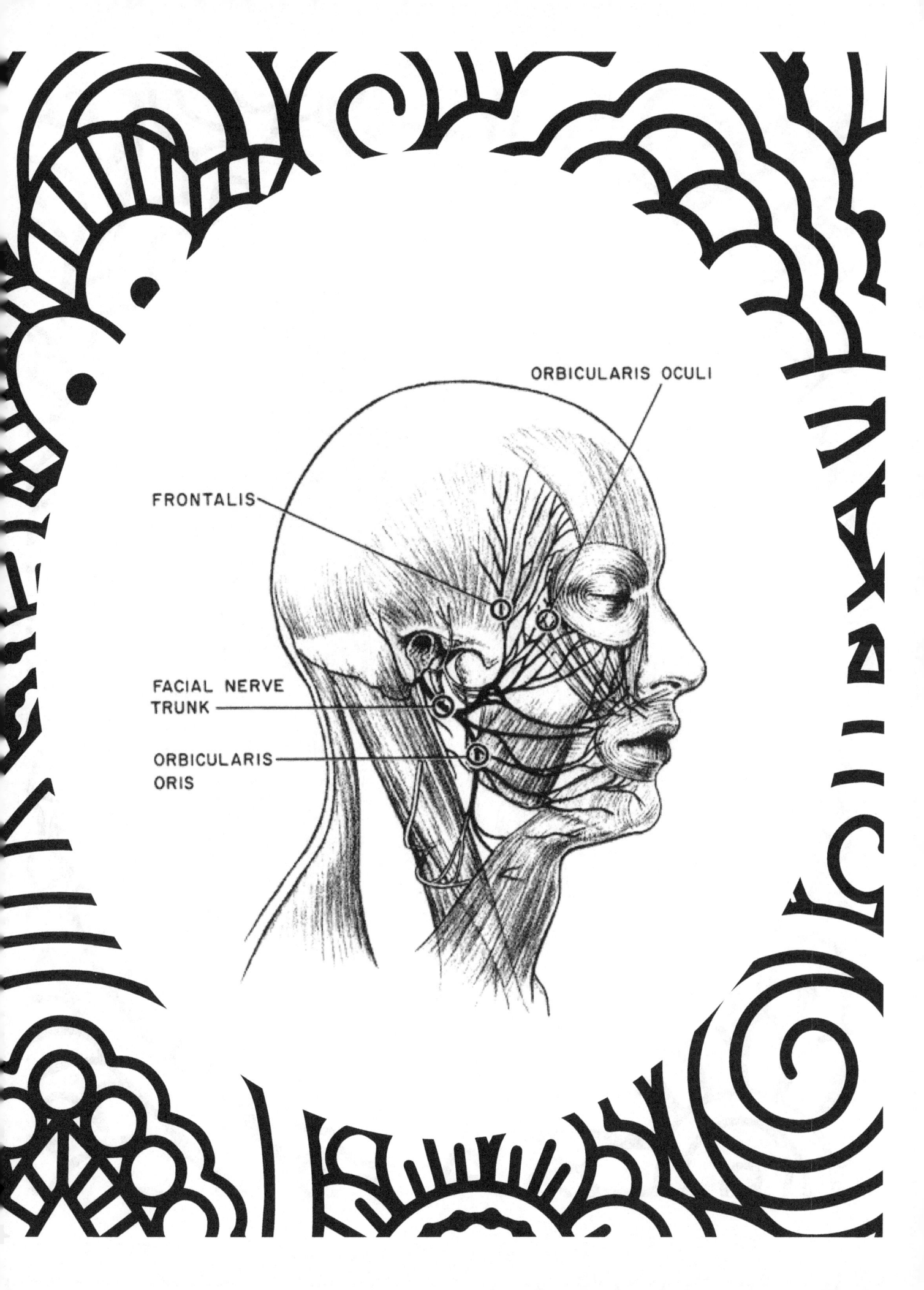

FRONTALIS

FACIAL NERVE TRUNK

ORBICULARIS ORIS

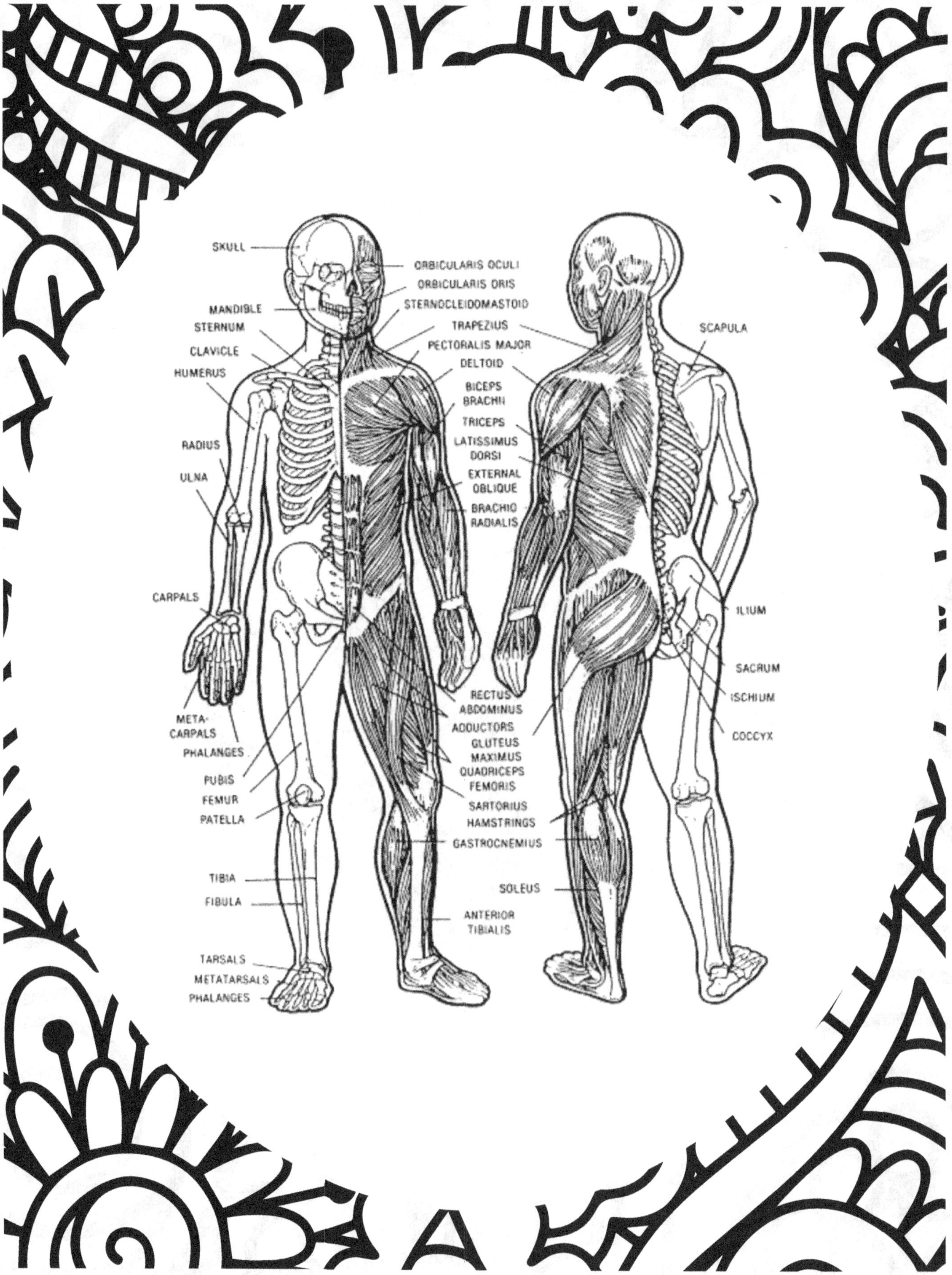

SKULL
ORBICULARIS OCULI
ORBICULARIS ORIS
MANDIBLE
STERNOCLEIDOMASTOID
STERNUM
TRAPEZIUS
SCAPULA
CLAVICLE
PECTORALIS MAJOR
HUMERUS
DELTOID
BICEPS BRACHII
TRICEPS
RADIUS
LATISSIMUS DORSI
ULNA
EXTERNAL OBLIQUE
BRACHIO RADIALIS
CARPALS
ILIUM
SACRUM
RECTUS ABDOMINUS
ISCHIUM
META-CARPALS
ADDUCTORS
COCCYX
PHALANGES
GLUTEUS MAXIMUS
QUADRICEPS FEMORIS
PUBIS
FEMUR
SARTORIUS
PATELLA
HAMSTRINGS
GASTROCNEMIUS
TIBIA
SOLEUS
FIBULA
ANTERIOR TIBIALIS
TARSALS
METATARSALS
PHALANGES

Human Muscles

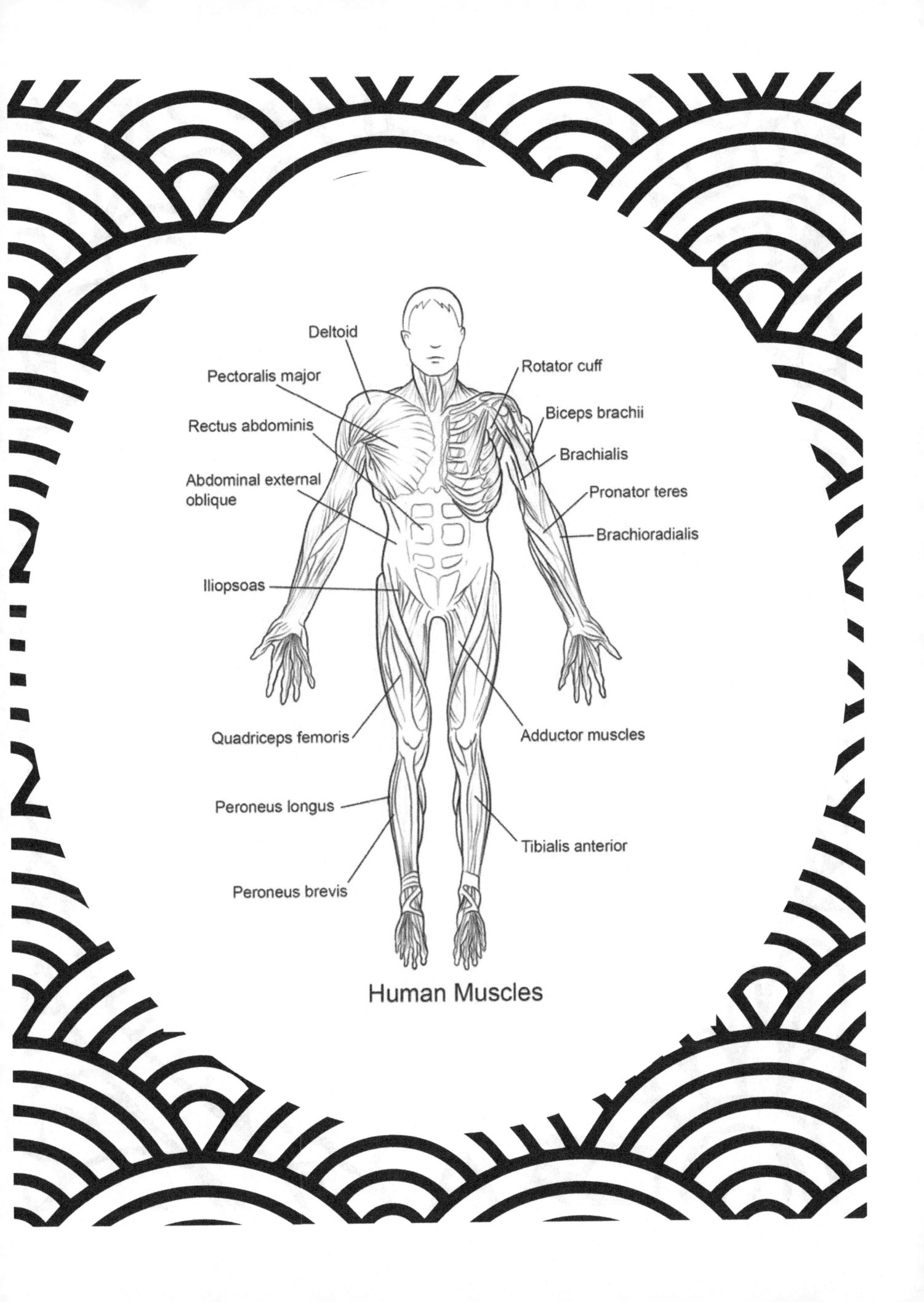

- Deltoid
- Pectoralis major
- Rectus abdominis
- Abdominal external oblique
- Iliopsoas
- Quadriceps femoris
- Peroneus longus
- Peroneus brevis
- Rotator cuff
- Biceps brachii
- Brachialis
- Pronator teres
- Brachioradialis
- Adductor muscles
- Tibialis anterior

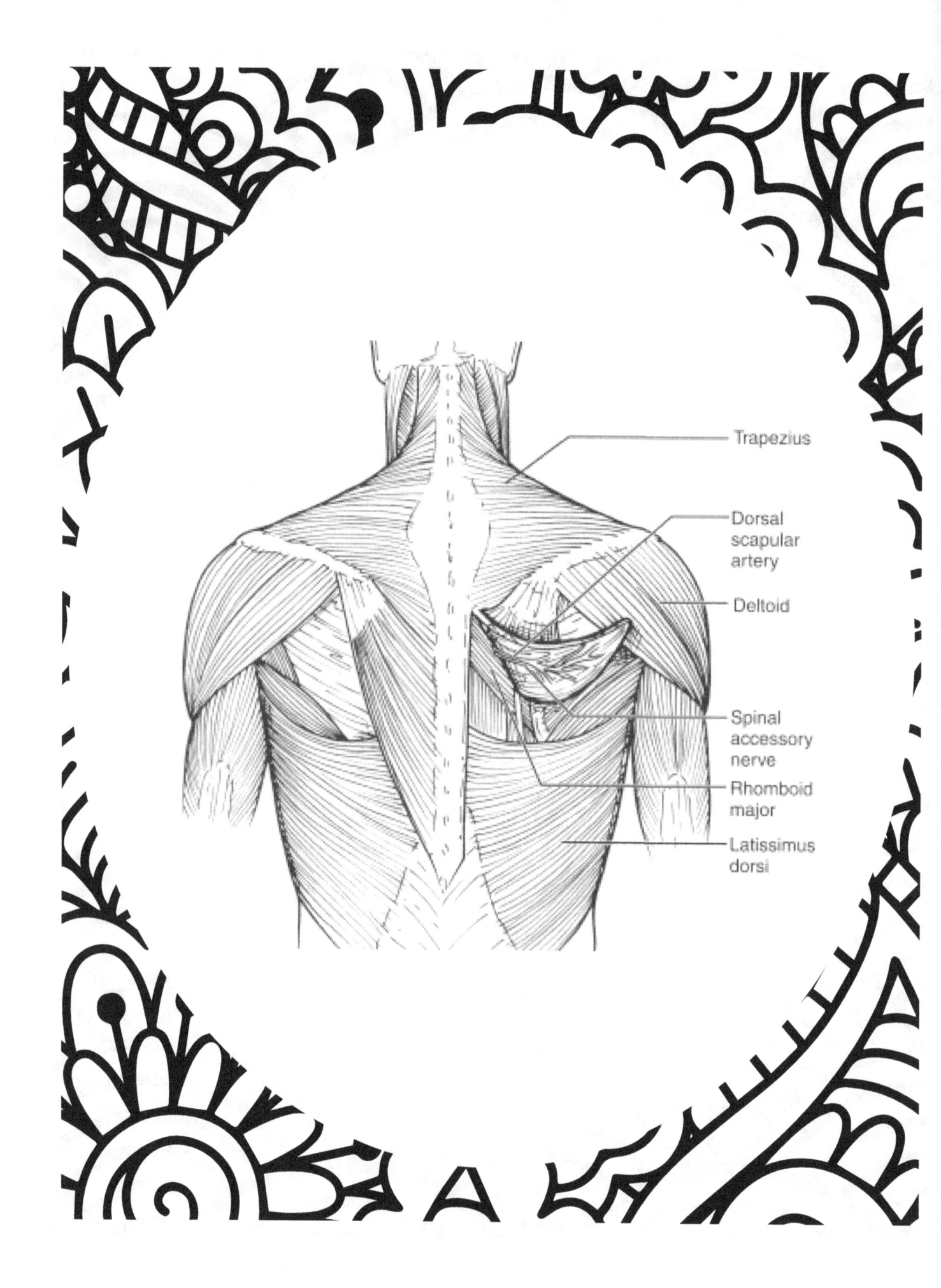

- Trapezius
- Dorsal scapular artery
- Deltoid
- Spinal accessory nerve
- Rhomboid major
- Latissimus dorsi

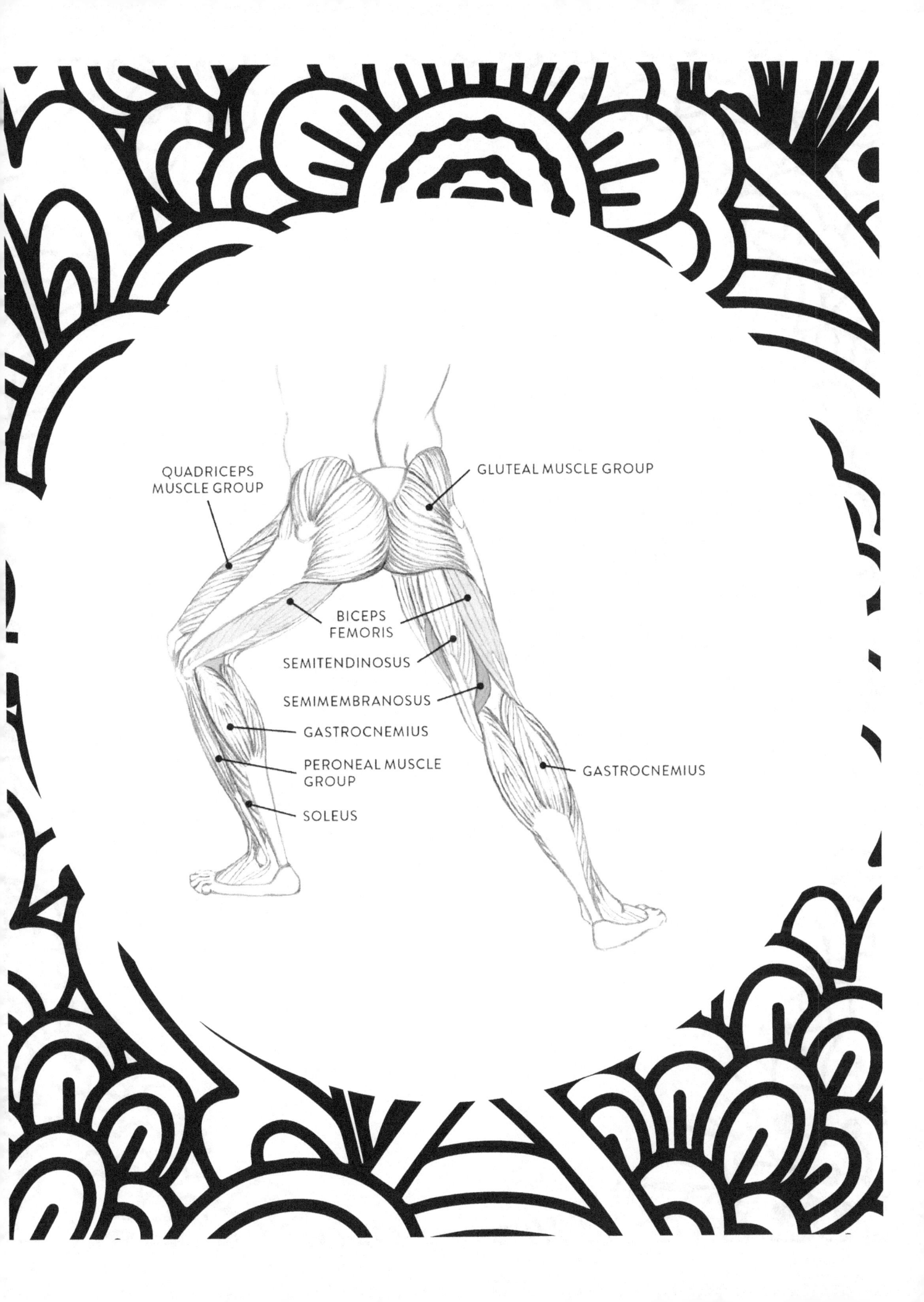

- QUADRICEPS MUSCLE GROUP
- GLUTEAL MUSCLE GROUP
- BICEPS FEMORIS
- SEMITENDINOSUS
- SEMIMEMBRANOSUS
- GASTROCNEMIUS
- PERONEAL MUSCLE GROUP
- SOLEUS
- GASTROCNEMIUS

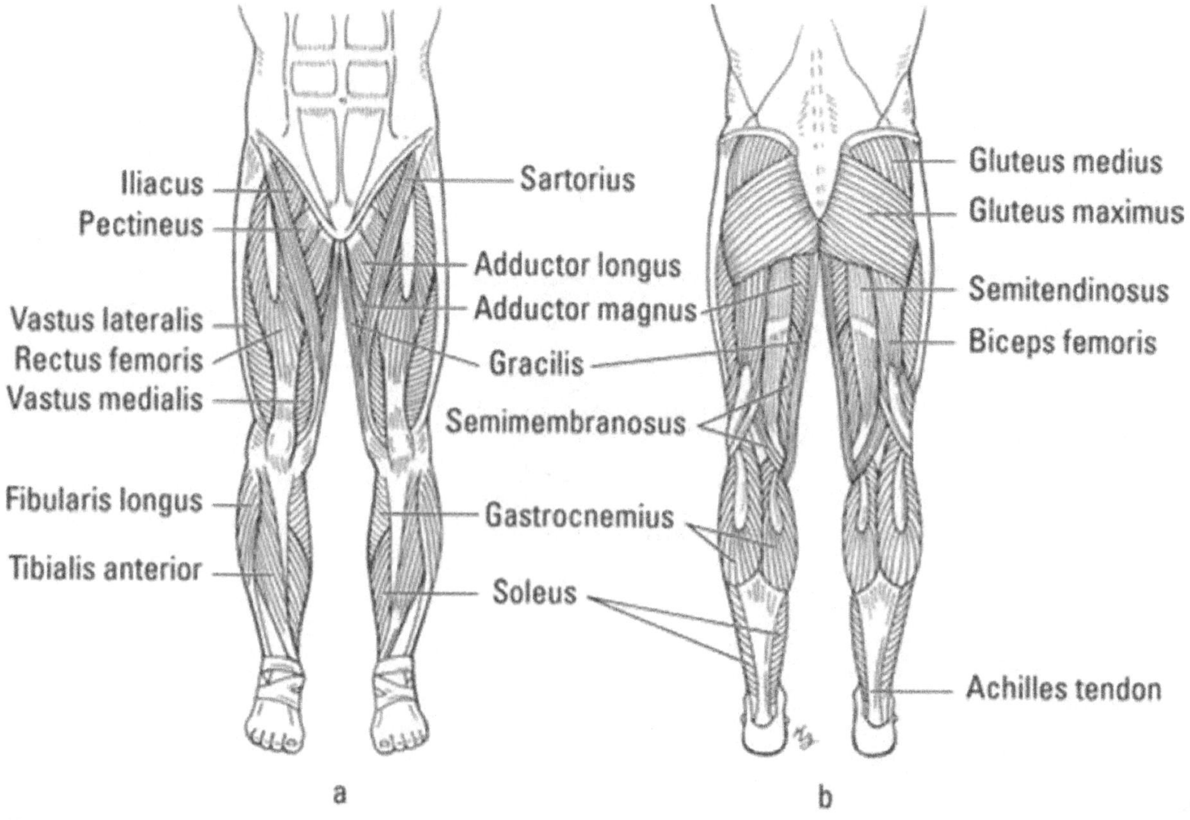
Iliacus
Pectineus
Vastus lateralis
Rectus femoris
Vastus medialis
Fibularis longus
Tibialis anterior
Sartorius
Adductor longus
Adductor magnus
Gracilis
Semimembranosus
Gastrocnemius
Soleus
Gluteus medius
Gluteus maximus
Semitendinosus
Biceps femoris
Achilles tendon
a
b

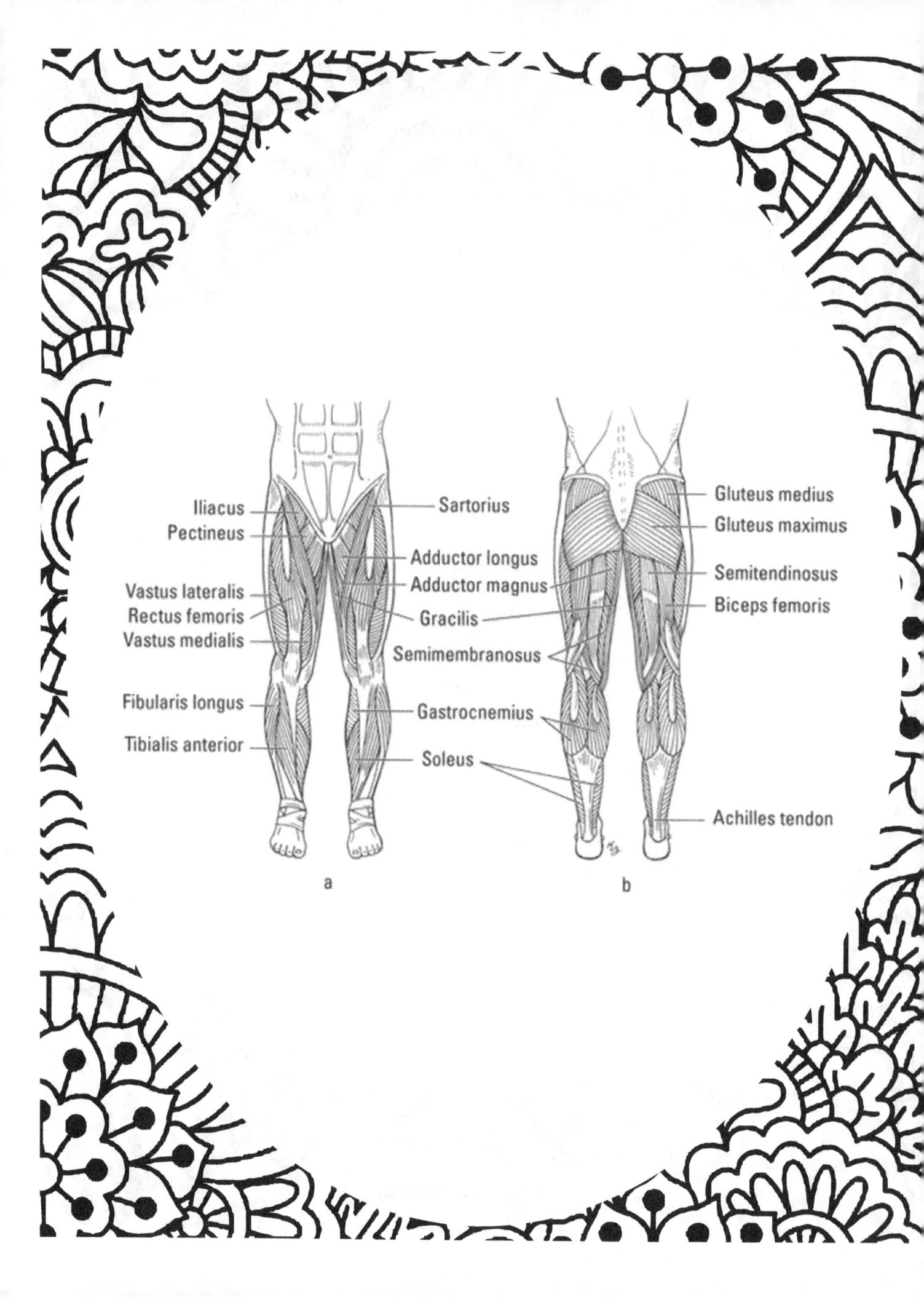

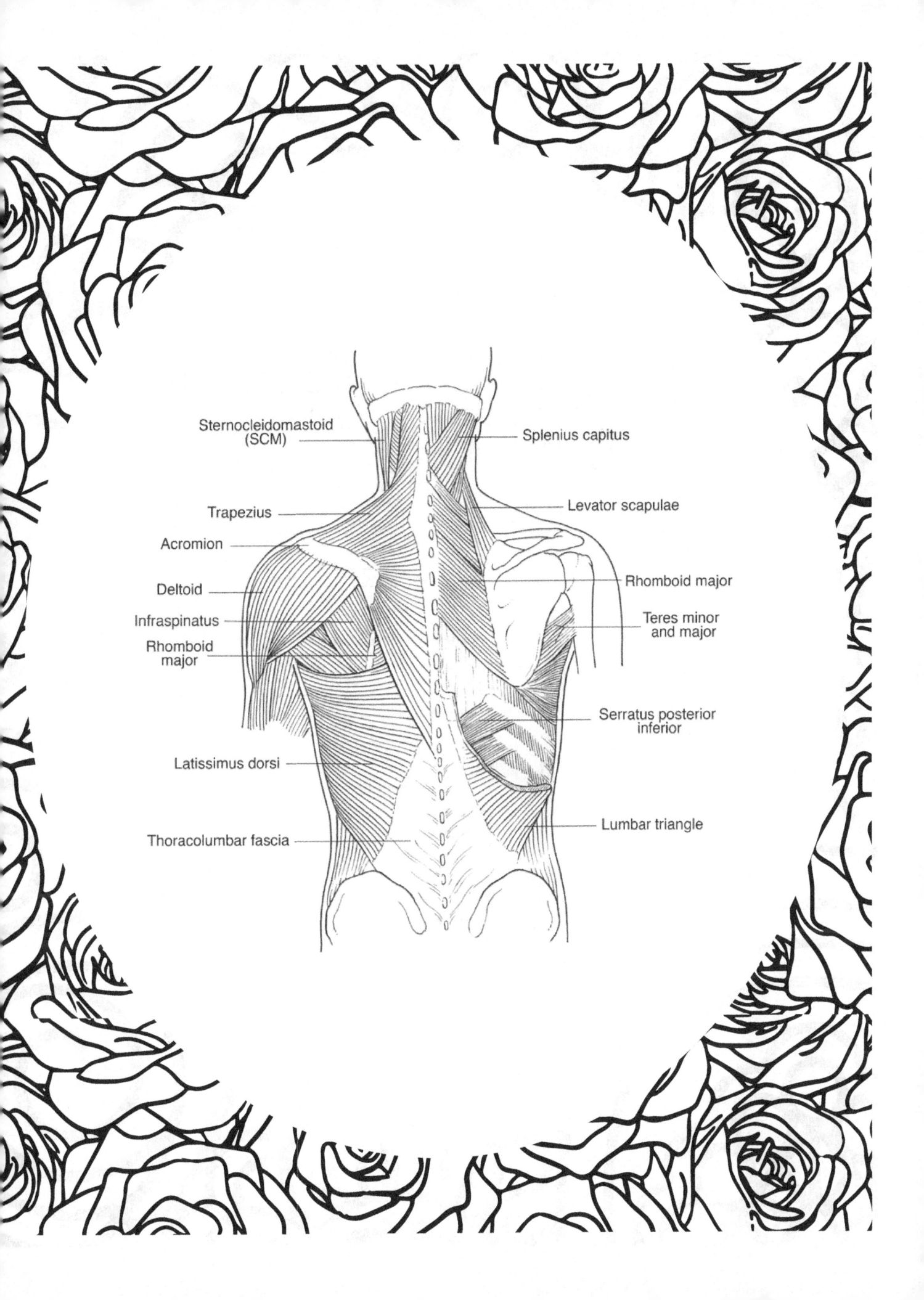

- Sternocleidomastoid (SCM)
- Splenius capitus
- Trapezius
- Levator scapulae
- Acromion
- Deltoid
- Rhomboid major
- Infraspinatus
- Teres minor and major
- Rhomboid major
- Serratus posterior inferior
- Latissimus dorsi
- Lumbar triangle
- Thoracolumbar fascia

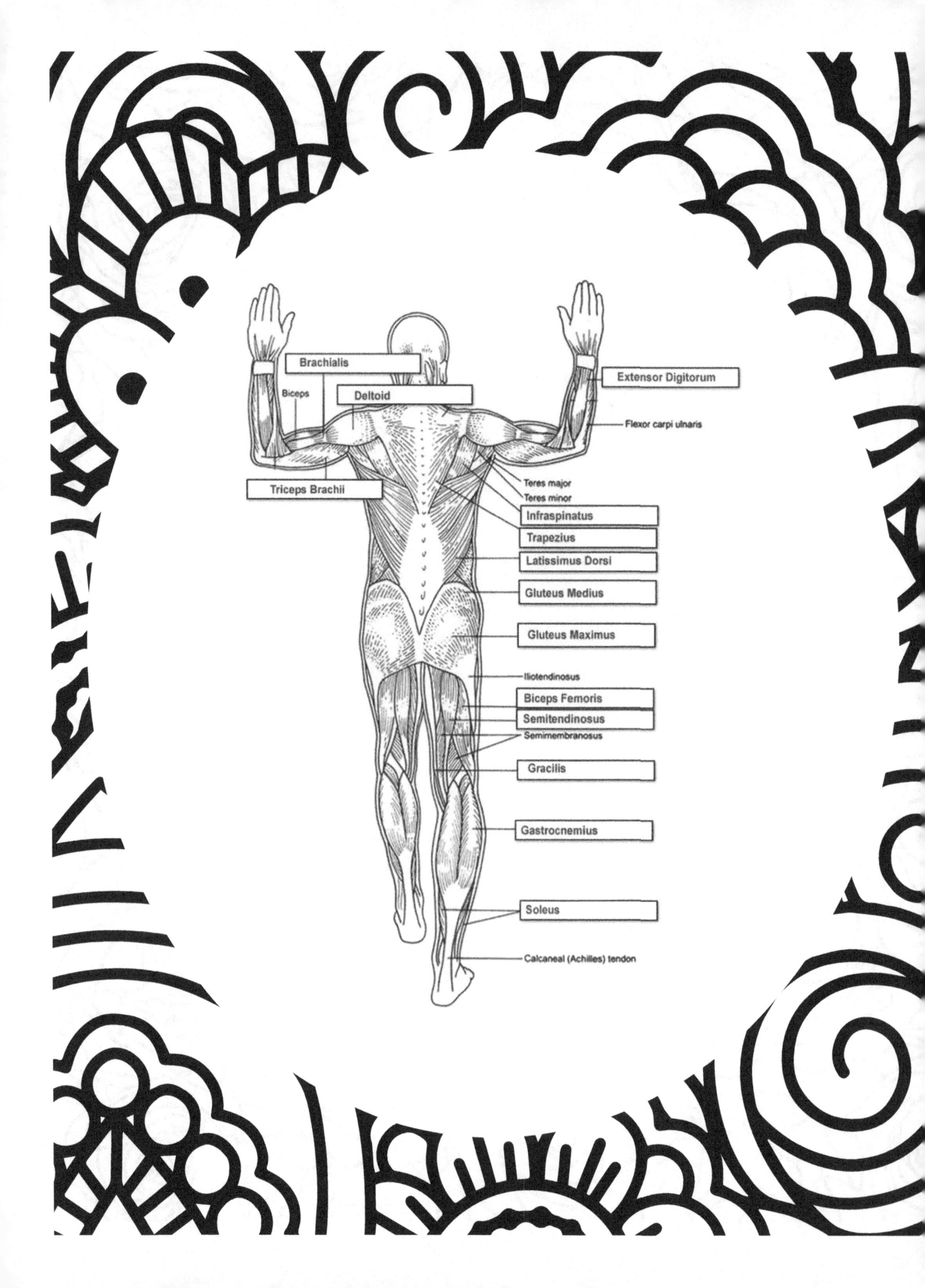

- Brachialis
- Biceps
- Deltoid
- Extensor Digitorum
- Flexor carpi ulnaris
- Triceps Brachii
- Teres major
- Teres minor
- Infraspinatus
- Trapezius
- Latissimus Dorsi
- Gluteus Medius
- Gluteus Maximus
- Iliotendinosus
- Biceps Femoris
- Semitendinosus
- Semimembranosus
- Gracilis
- Gastrocnemius
- Soleus
- Calcaneal (Achilles) tendon

Region 1: submental

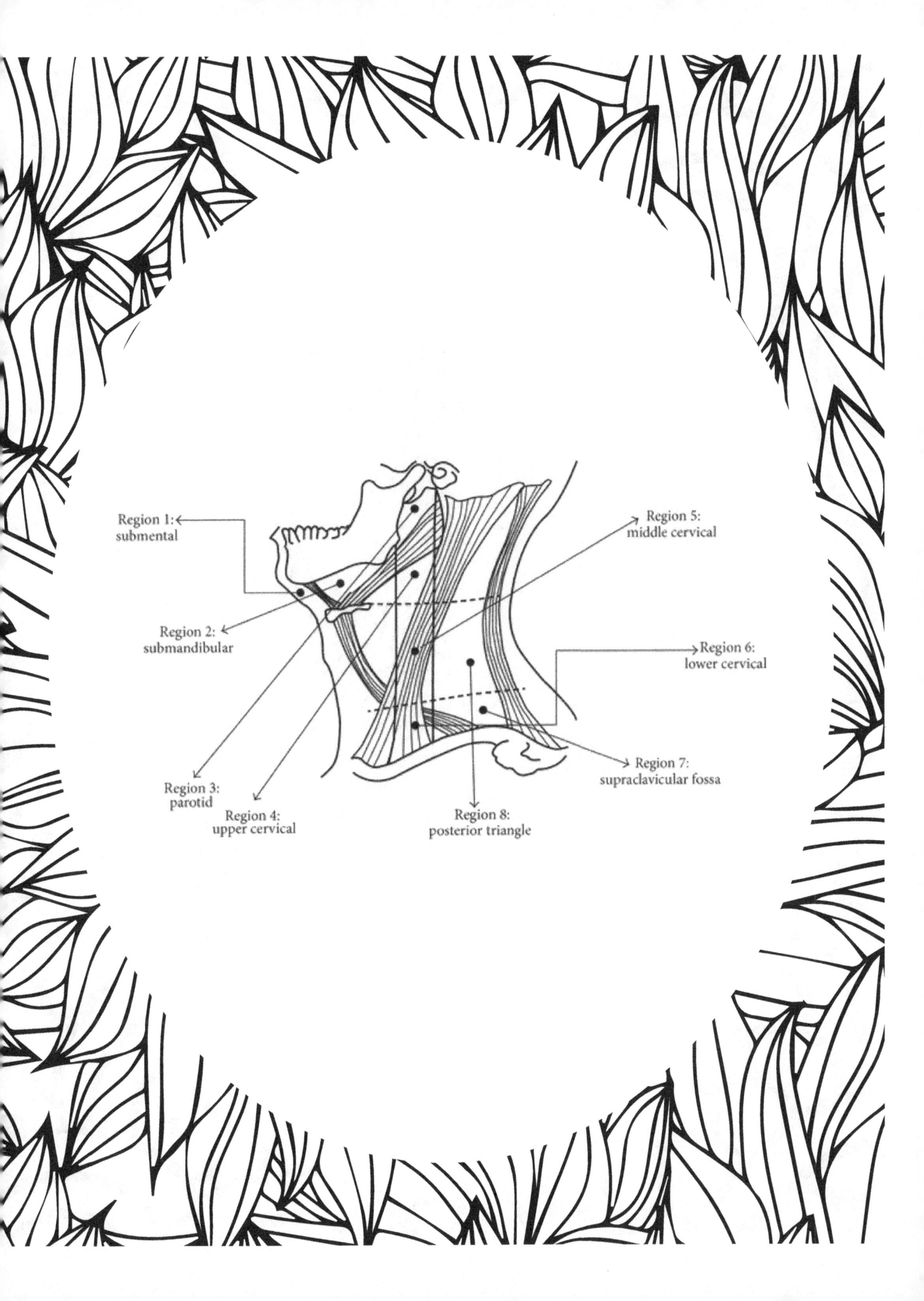

Region 2: submandibular

Region 3: parotid

Region 4: upper cervical

Region 5: middle cervical

Region 6: lower cervical

Region 7: supraclavicular fossa

Region 8: posterior triangle

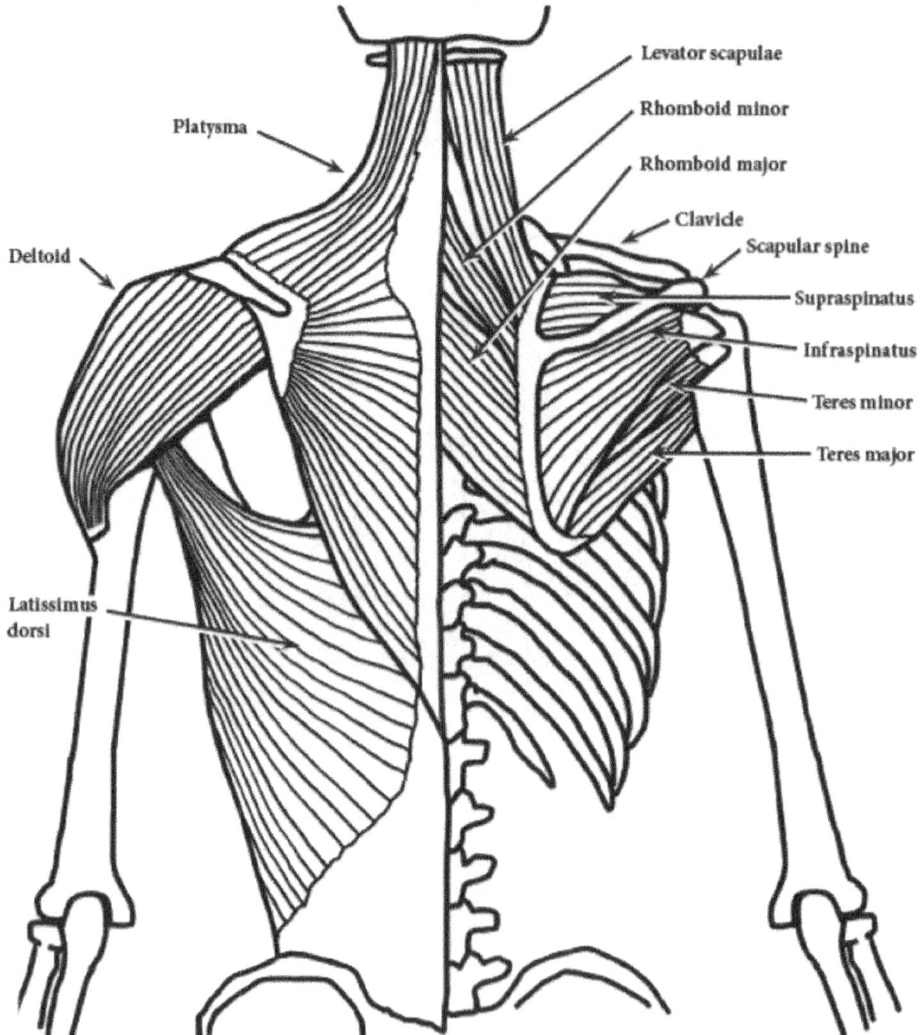

Levator scapulae
Rhomboid minor
Platysma
Rhomboid major
Clavicle
Deltoid
Scapular spine
Supraspinatus
Infraspinatus
Teres minor
Teres major
Latissimus
dorsi

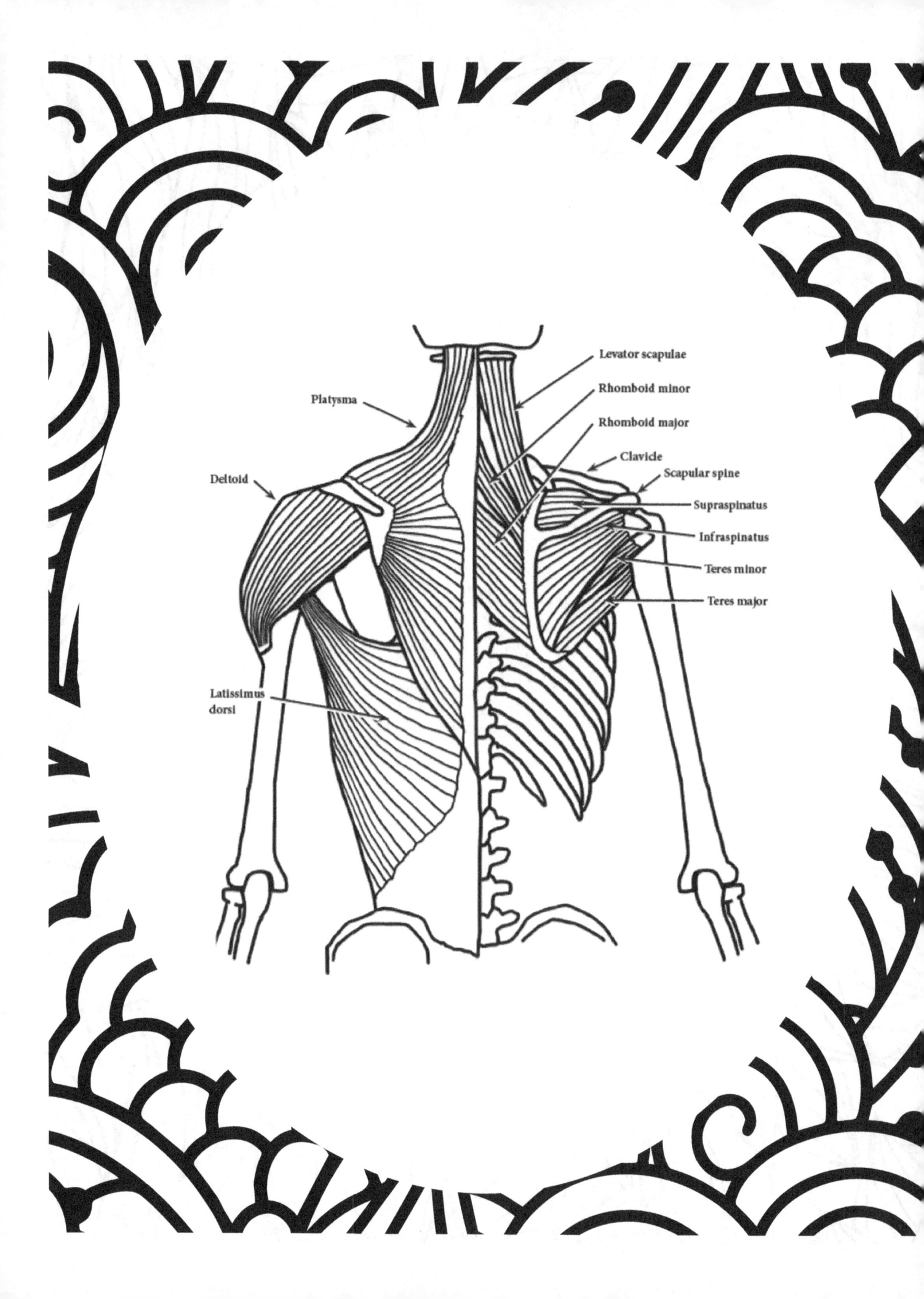

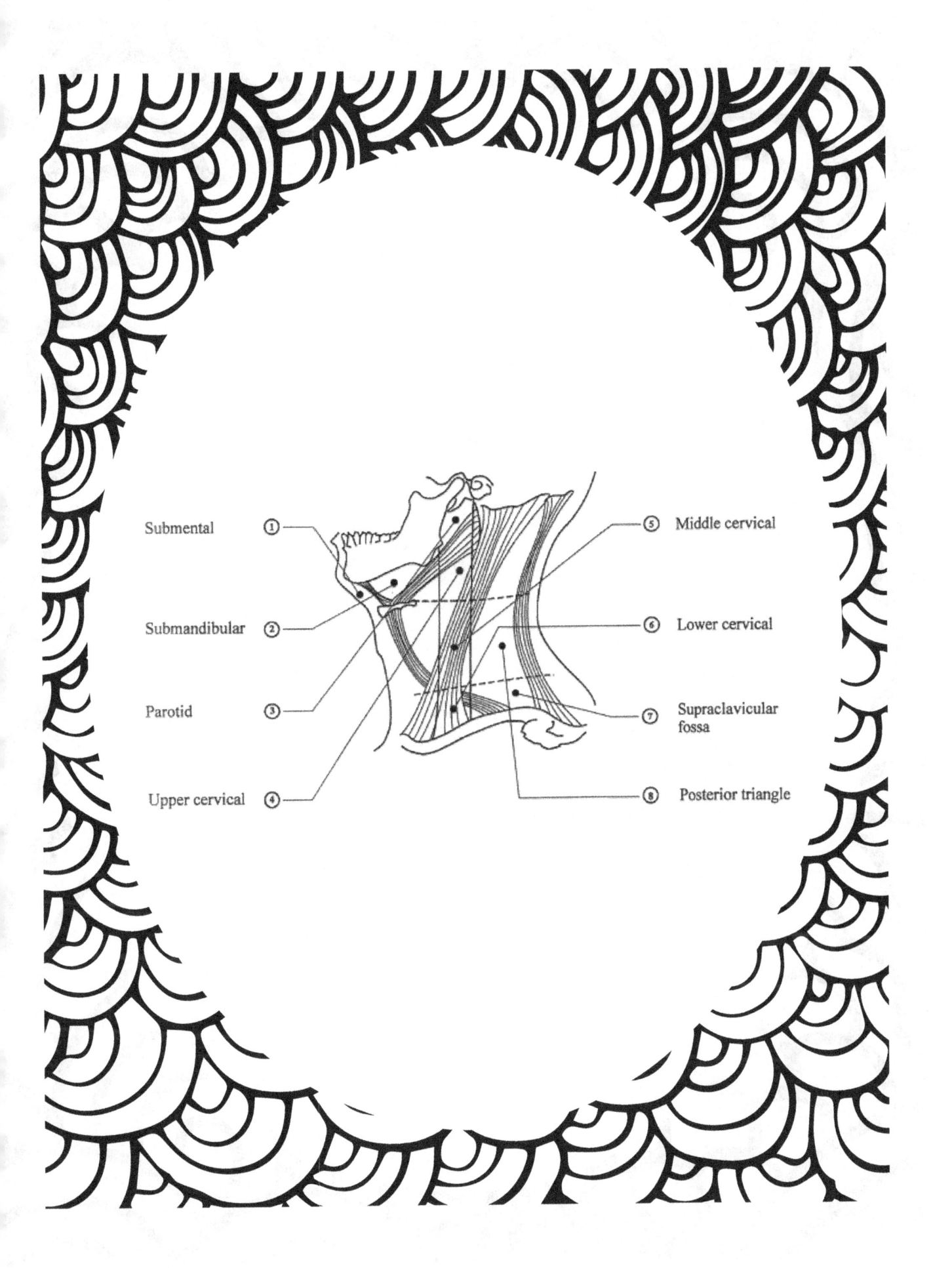

Submental	①	⑤	Middle cervical
Submandibular	②	⑥	Lower cervical
Parotid	③	⑦	Supraclavicular fossa
Upper cervical	④	⑧	Posterior triangle

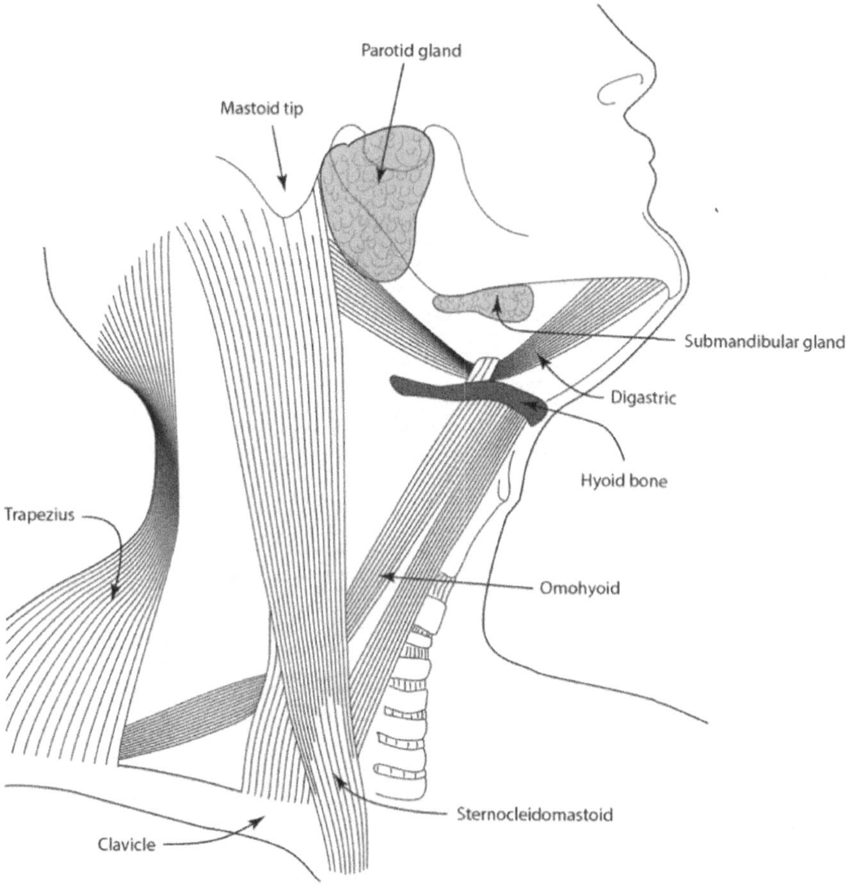
Parotid gland
Mastoid tip
Submandibular gland
Digastric
Hyoid bone
Trapezius
Omohyoid
Sternocleidomastoid
Clavicle

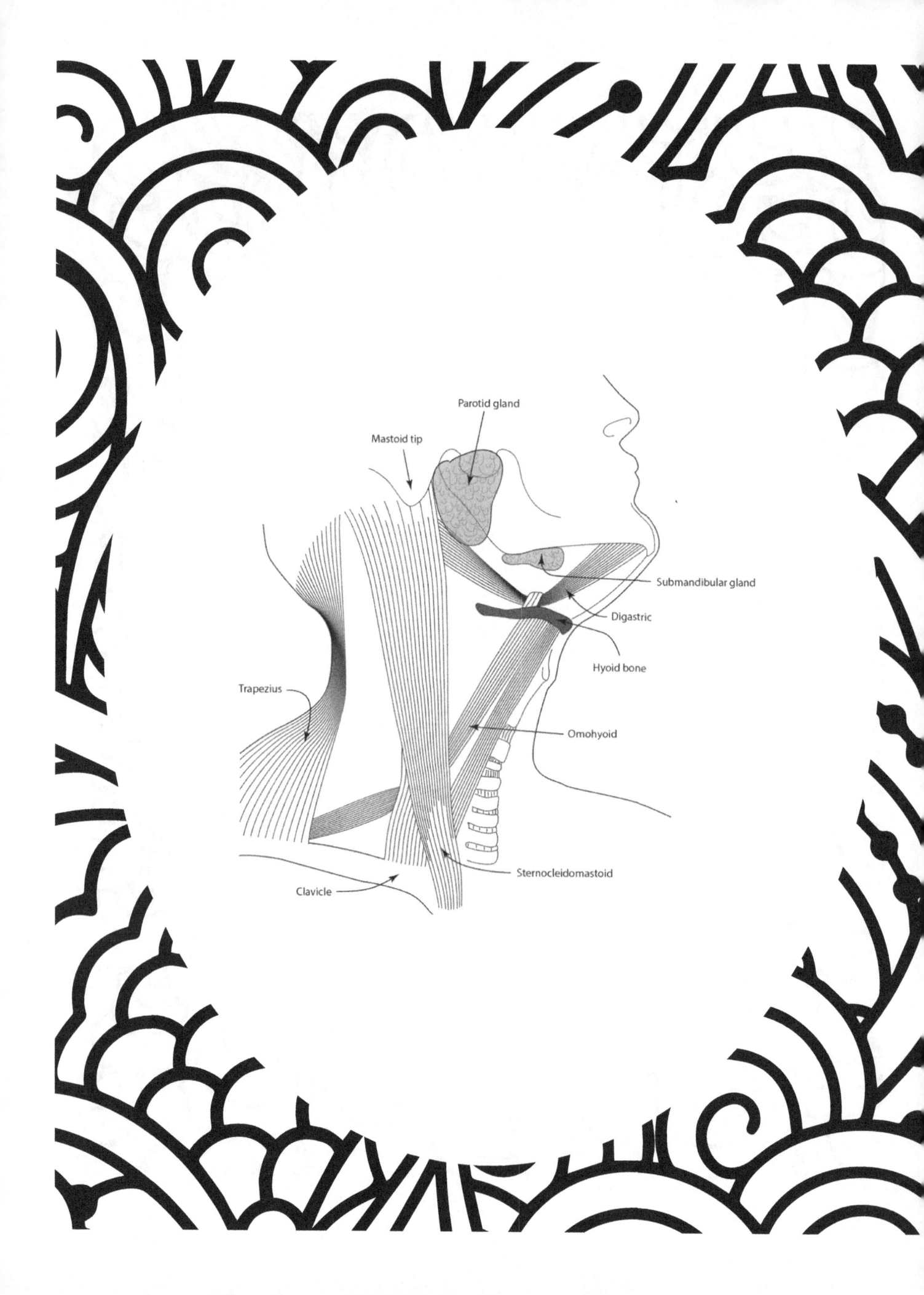

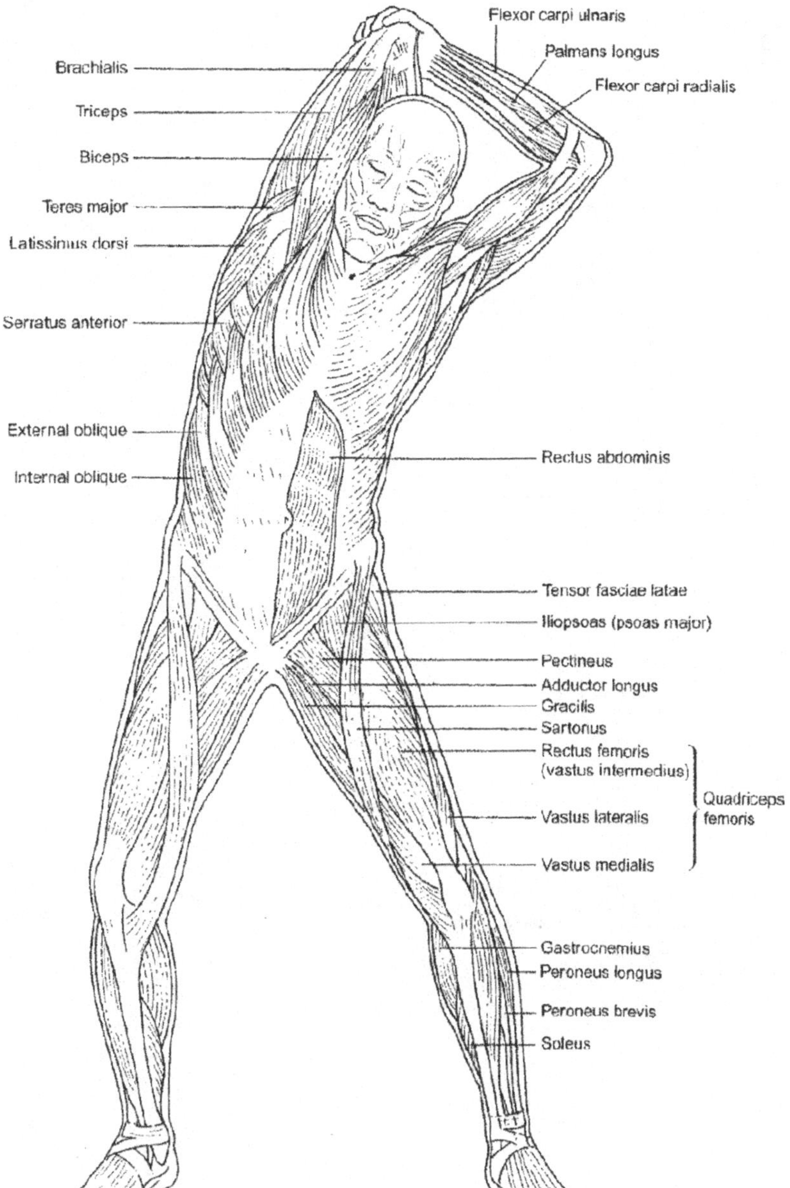

Flexor carpi ulnaris
Palmans longus
Flexor carpi radialis
Brachialis
Triceps
Biceps
Teres major
Latissinius dorsi
Serratus anterior
External oblique
Internal oblique
Rectus abdominis
Tensor fasciae latae
Iliopsoas (psoas major)
Pectineus
Adductor longus
Gracilis
Sartonus
Rectus femoris
(vastus intermedius)
Vastus lateralis
Vastus medialis
Quadriceps
femoris
Gastrocnemius
Peroneus longus
Peroneus brevis
Soleus

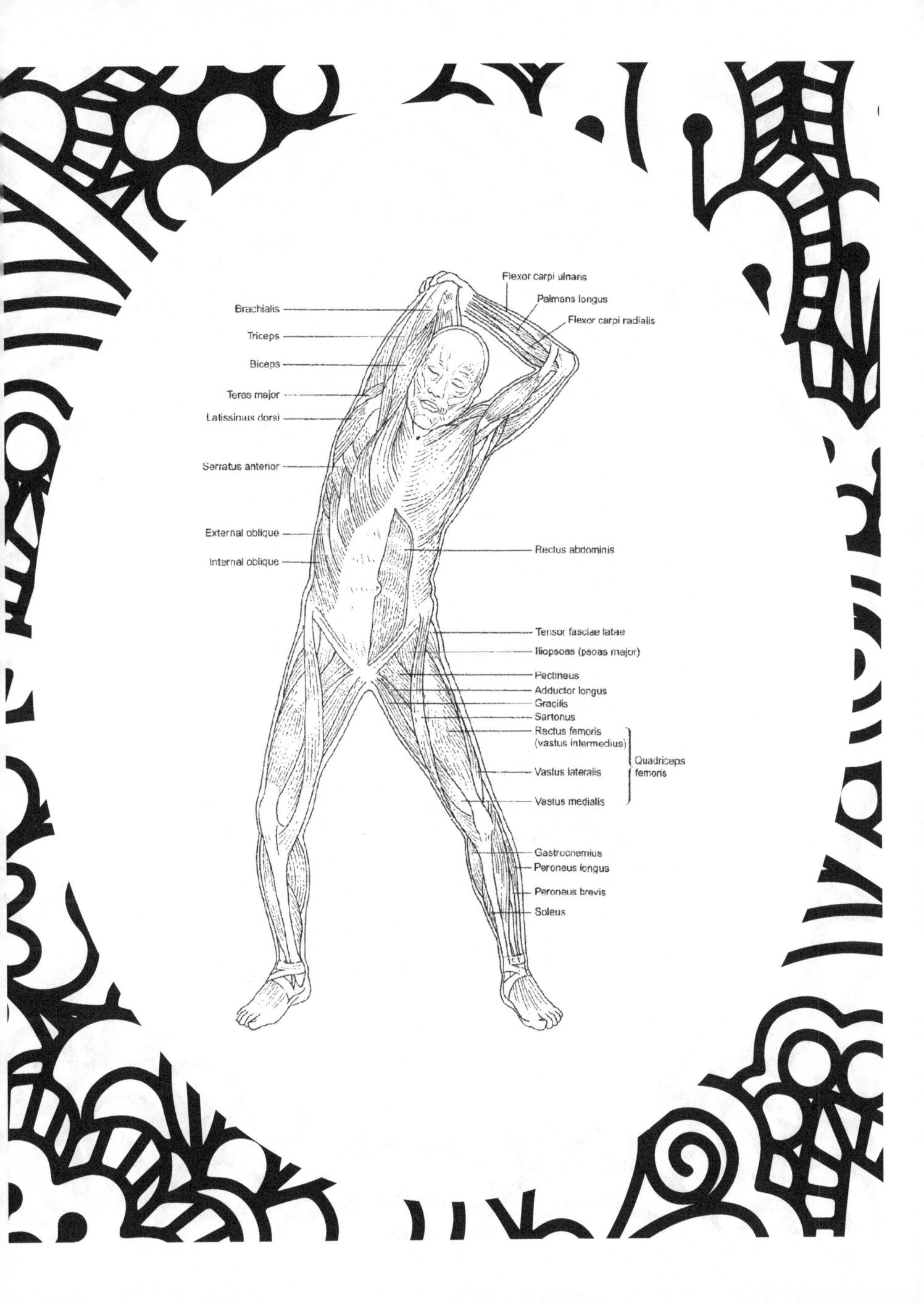

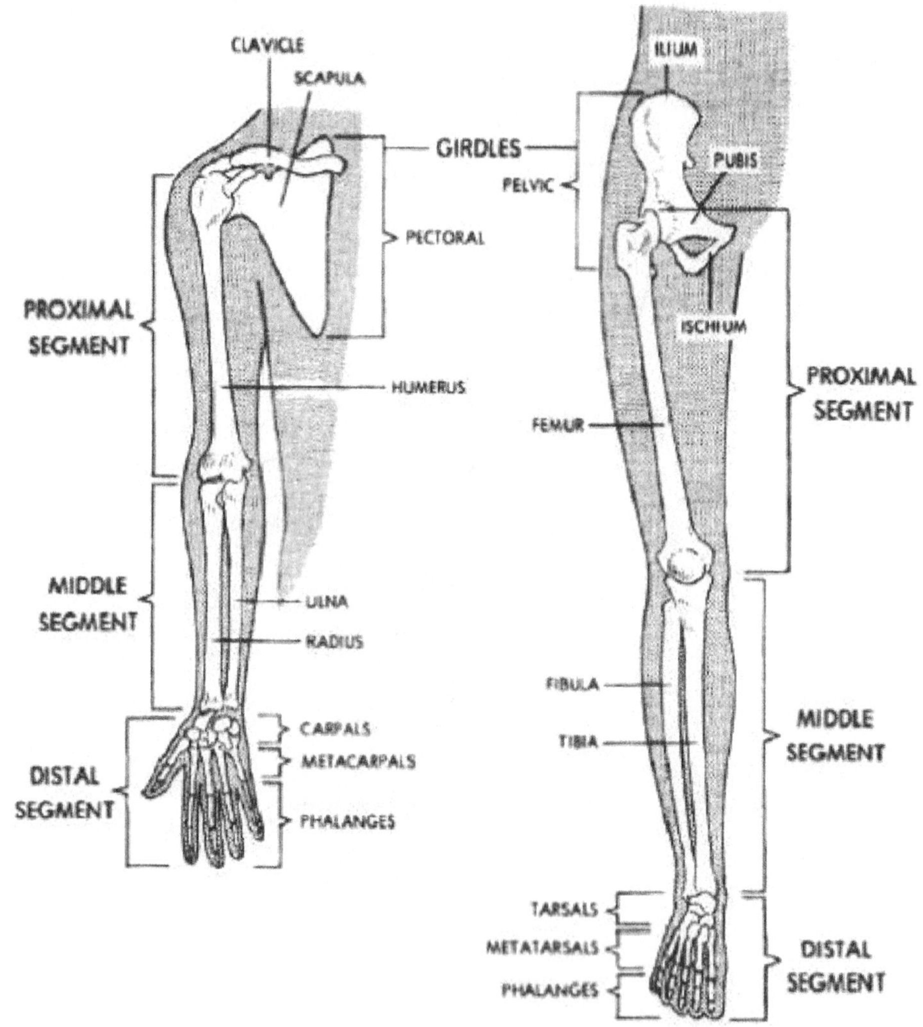

CLAVICLE
SCAPULA
GIRDLES
PELVIC
PECTORAL
ILIUM
PUBIS
ISCHIUM
PROXIMAL SEGMENT
HUMERUS
PROXIMAL SEGMENT
FEMUR
MIDDLE SEGMENT
ULNA
RADIUS
FIBULA
TIBIA
MIDDLE SEGMENT
CARPALS
METACARPALS
DISTAL SEGMENT
PHALANGES
TARSALS
METATARSALS
PHALANGES
DISTAL SEGMENT

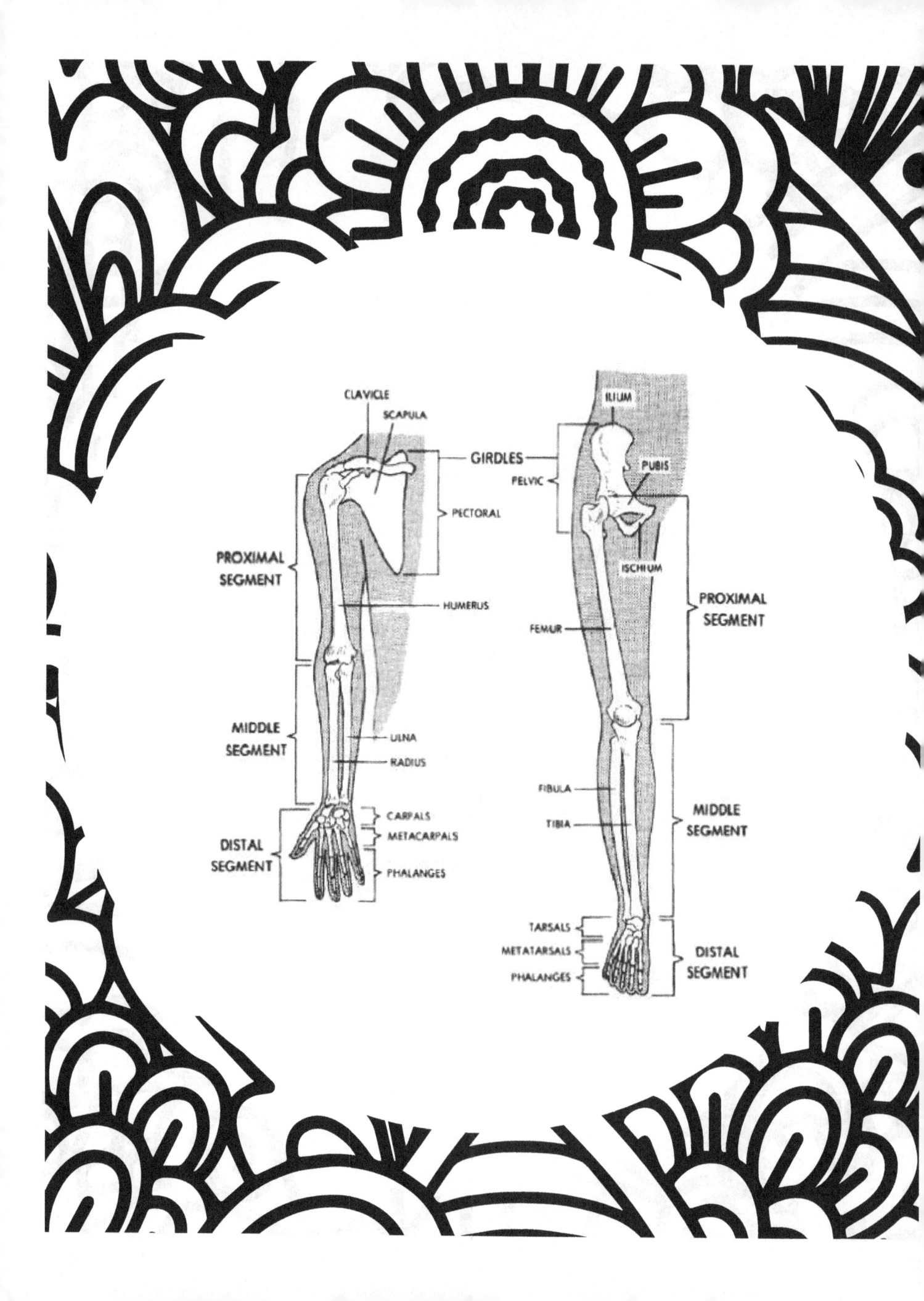

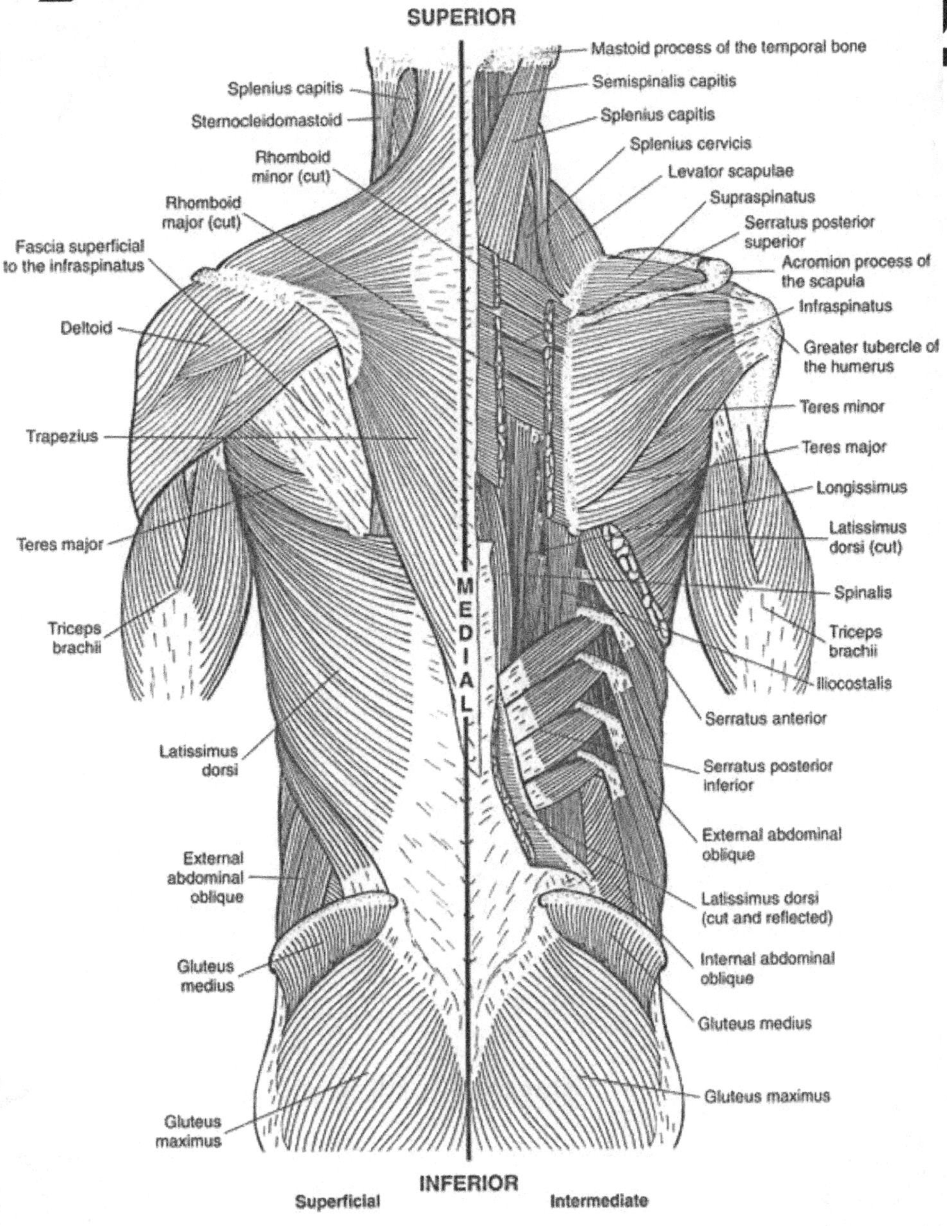

SUPERIOR
Mastoid process of the temporal bone
Splenius capitis
Semispinalis capitis
Sternocleidomastoid
Splenius capitis
Splenius cervicis
Rhomboid minor (cut)
Levator scapulae
Supraspinatus
Rhomboid major (cut)
Serratus posterior superior
Fascia superficial to the infraspinatus
Acromion process of the scapula
Infraspinatus
Deltoid
Greater tubercle of the humerus
Teres minor
Trapezius
Teres major
Longissimus
Teres major
Latissimus dorsi (cut)
MEDIAL
Spinalis
Triceps brachii
Triceps brachii
Iliocostalis
Serratus anterior
Latissimus dorsi
Serratus posterior inferior
External abdominal oblique
External abdominal oblique
Latissimus dorsi (cut and reflected)
Gluteus medius
Internal abdominal oblique
Gluteus medius
Gluteus maximus
Gluteus maximus
INFERIOR
Superficial
Intermediate

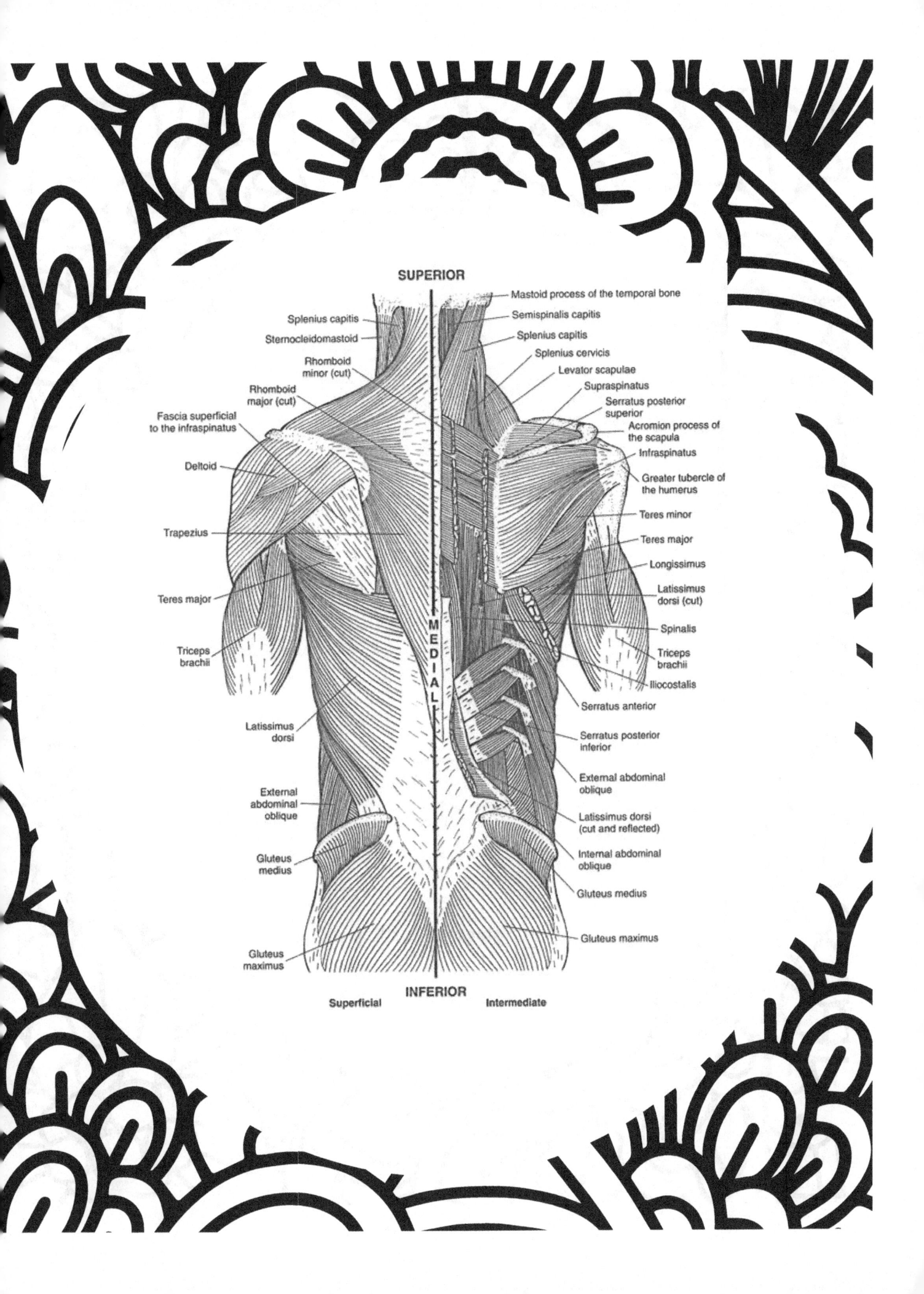

Human Muscles

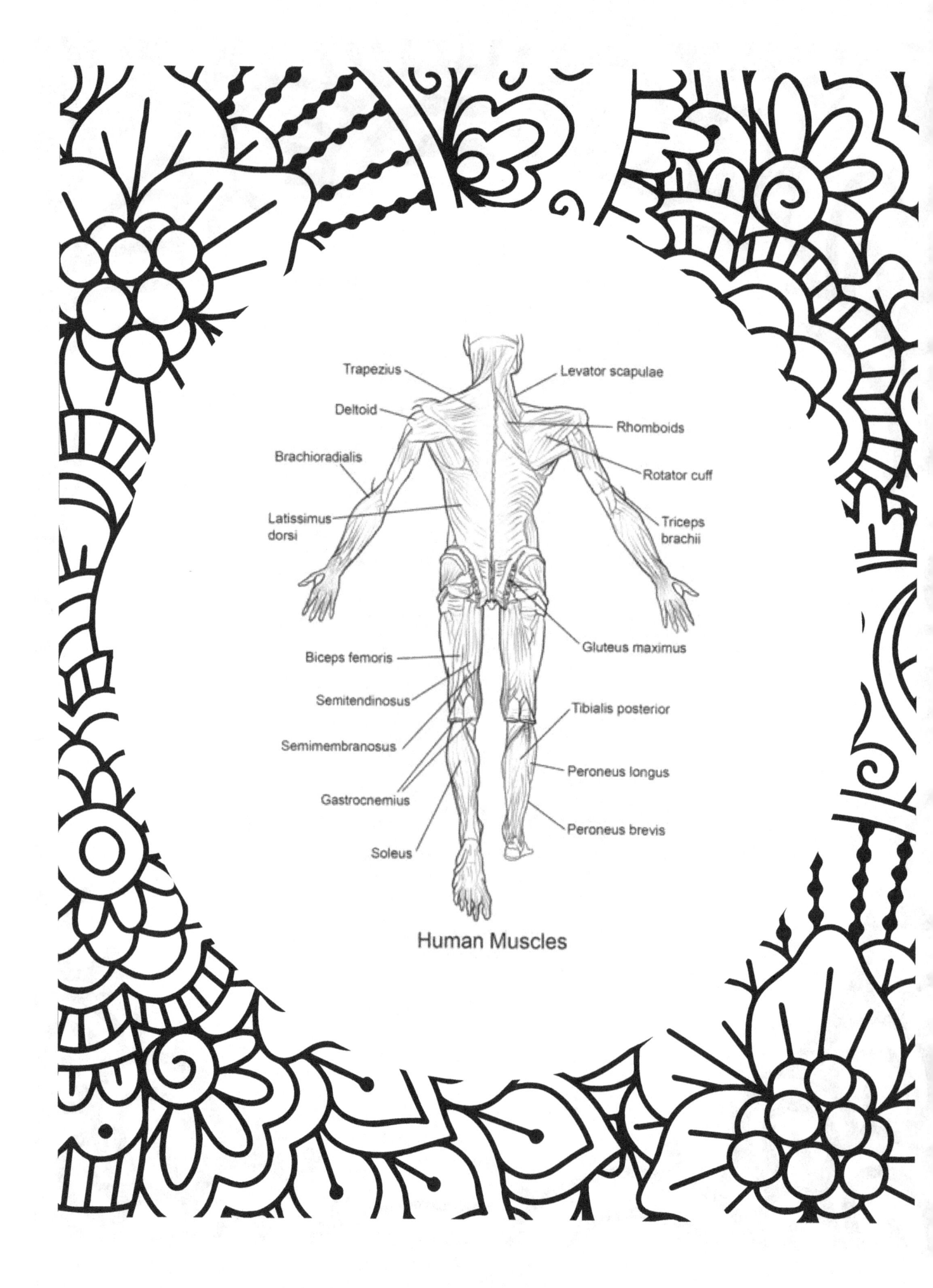

- Trapezius
- Levator scapulae
- Deltoid
- Rhomboids
- Brachioradialis
- Rotator cuff
- Latissimus dorsi
- Triceps brachii
- Gluteus maximus
- Biceps femoris
- Semitendinosus
- Tibialis posterior
- Semimembranosus
- Peroneus longus
- Gastrocnemius
- Peroneus brevis
- Soleus

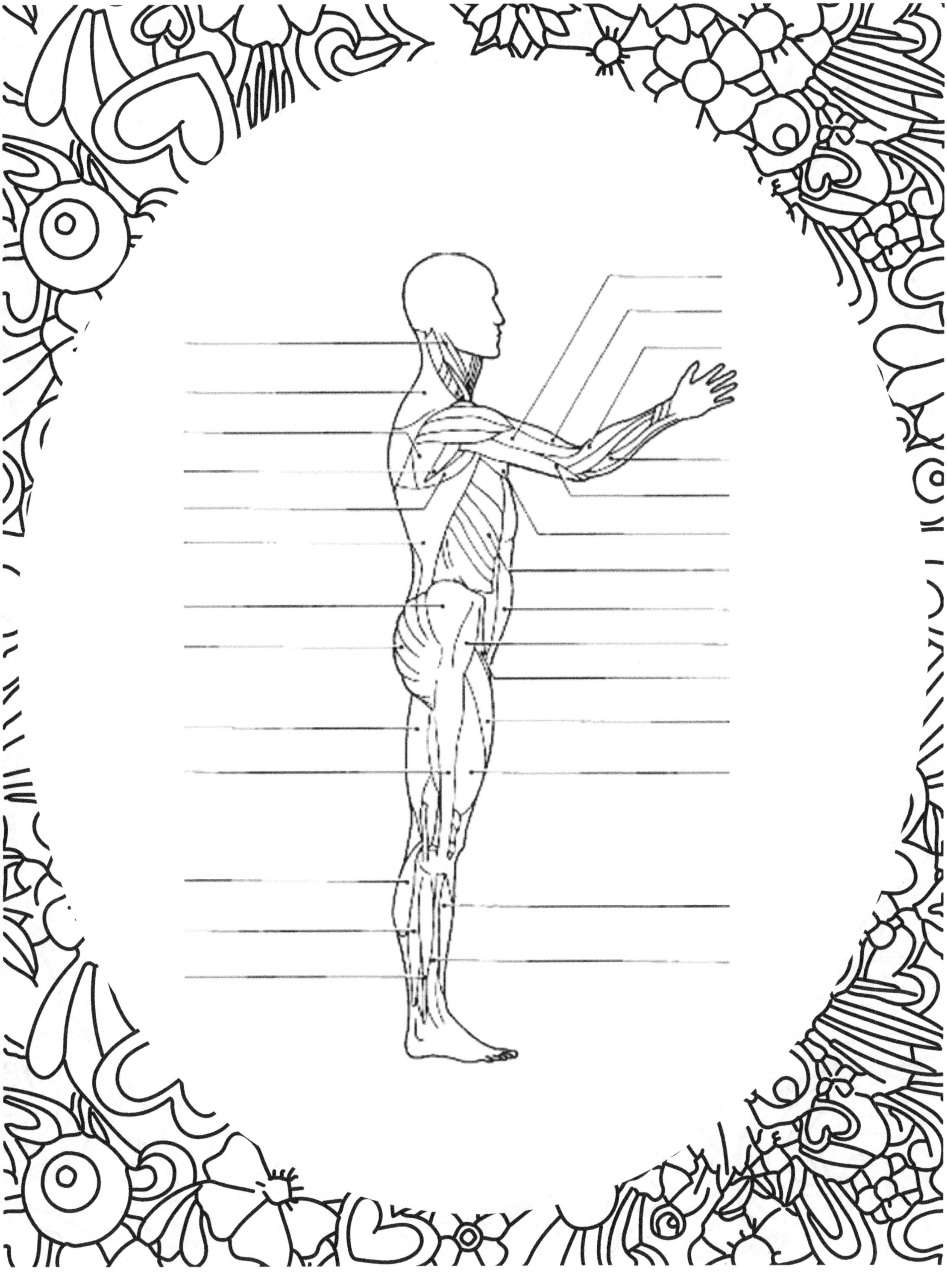

The Main Anterior Muscles of the Human body

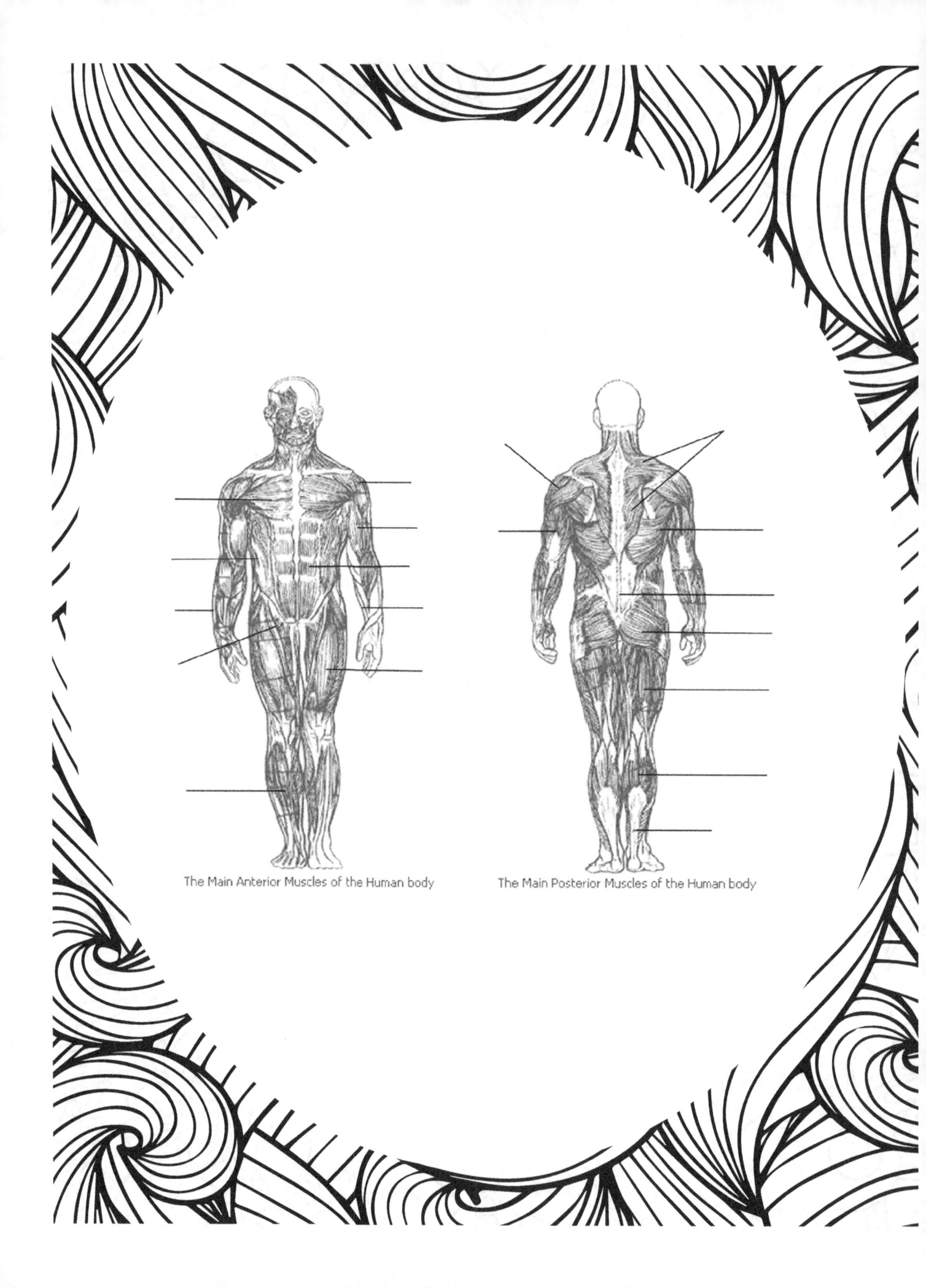

The Main Posterior Muscles of the Human body

Muscular System: Anterior

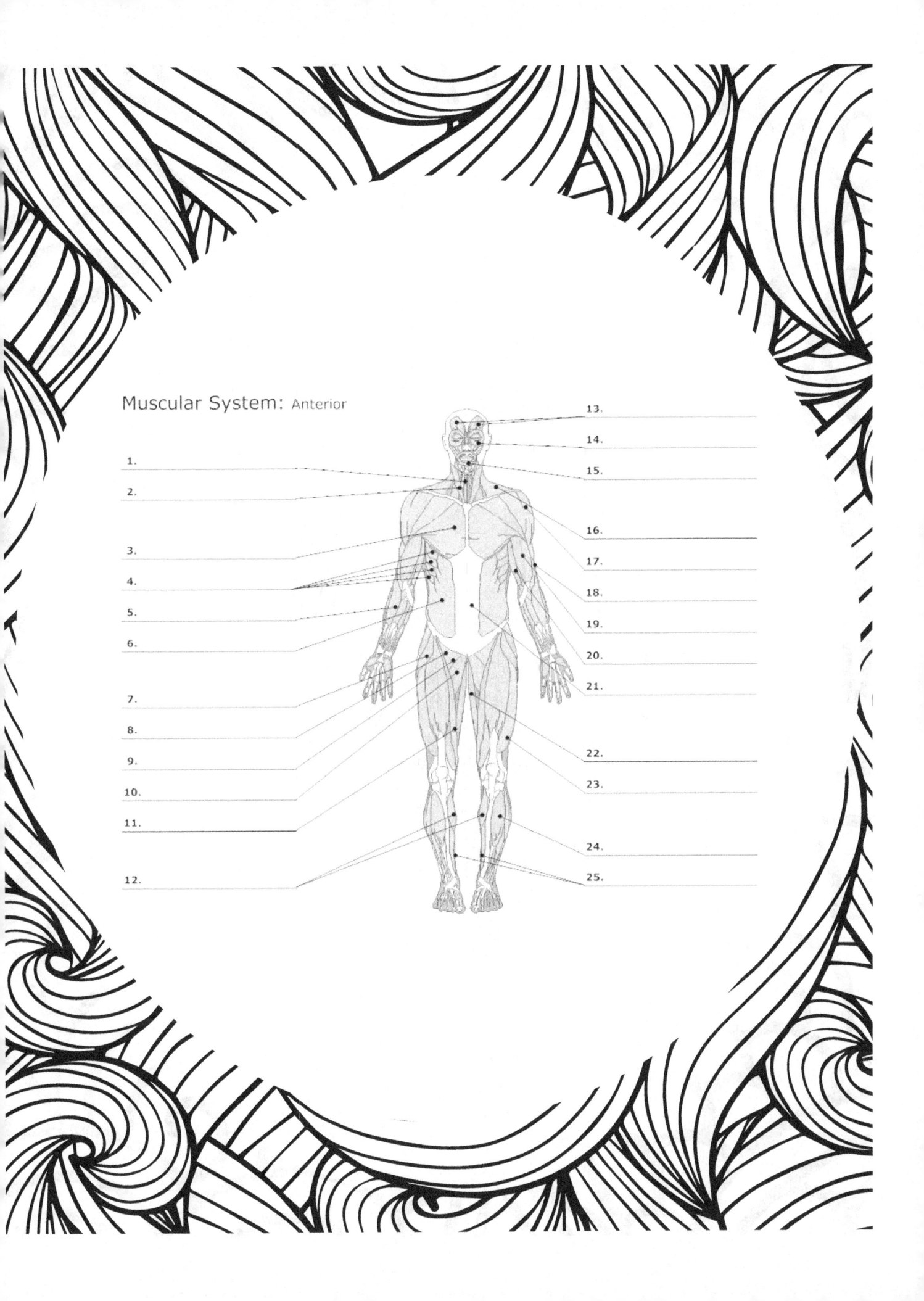

1.
2.
3.
4.
5.
6.
7.
8.
9.
10.
11.
12.
13.
14.
15.
16.
17.
18.
19.
20.
21.
22.
23.
24.
25.

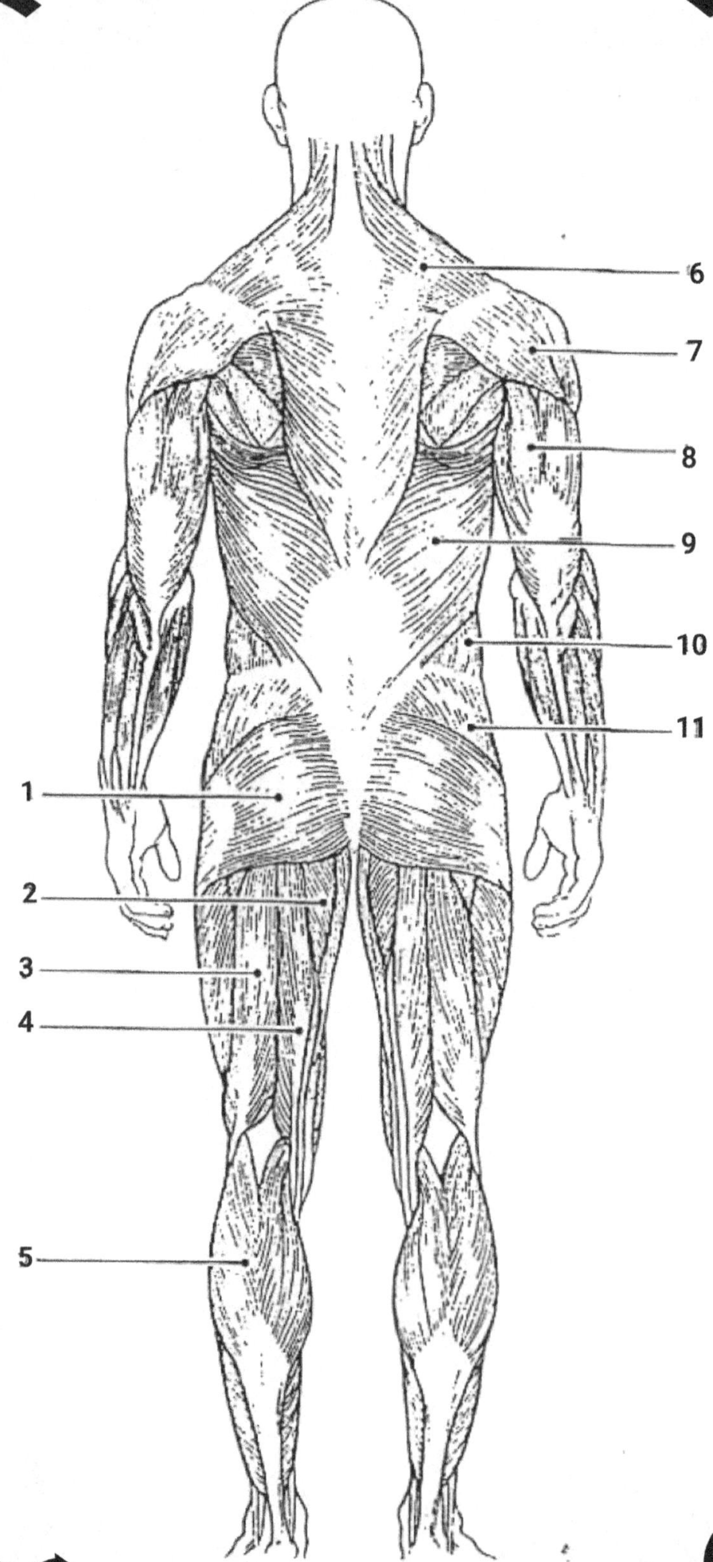

6
7
8
9
10
11
1
2
3
4
5

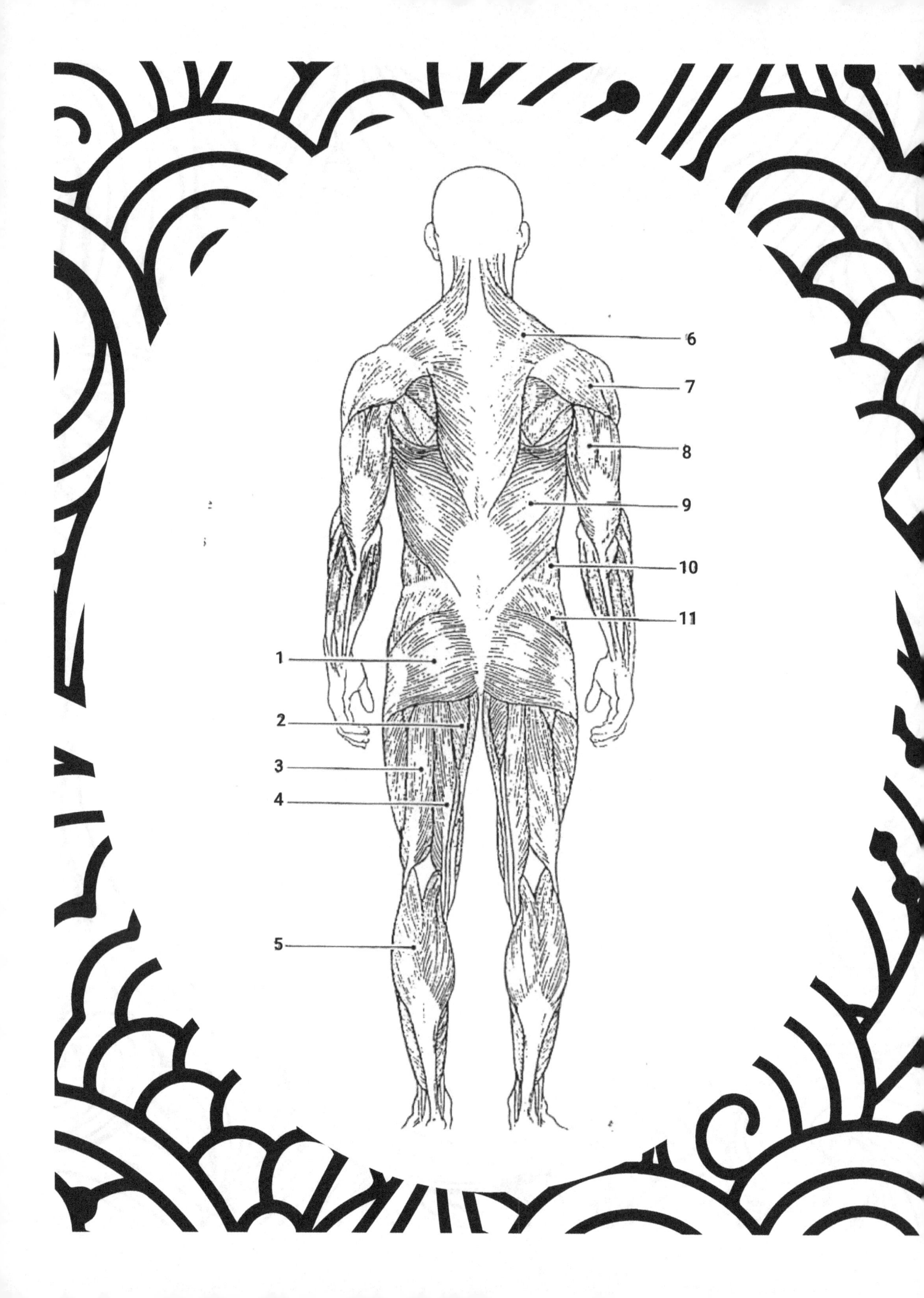